Total Revision:
Ear, Nose and Throat

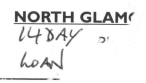

PASTEST
Dedicated to your success

Total Revision:
Ear, Nose and Throat

P Séamus Phillips
MA, BM, MRCS, DO-HNS
Specialist Registrar in Otolaryngology
South Thames Region, UK

and

Lydia Badia
FRCS (ORL-HNS)
Consultant Otolaryngologist
Royal National Throat, Nose and Ear Hospital, London, UK

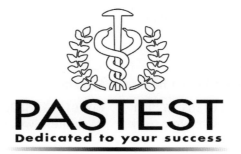

PASTEST
Dedicated to your success

© 2005 PasTest Ltd
Egerton Court
Parkgate Estate
Knutsford
Cheshire, WA16 8DX

Telephone: 01565 752000

First edition 2005

ISBN: 1 904 627 24 2

A catalogue record for this book is available from the British Library.

A percentage of the basic sciences practice questions in this title were previously published in *MRCS Core Modules: The Complete Test* and *MRCS System Modules: The Complete Test.*

The information contained within this book was obtained by the authors from reliable sources. However, while every effort has been made to ensure its accuracy, no responsibility for loss, damage or injury occasioned to any person acting or refraining from action as a result of information contained herein can be accepted by the publisher or the authors.

PasTest Revision Books and Intensive Courses

PasTest has been established in the field of postgraduate medical education since 1972, providing revision books and intensive study courses for doctors preparing for their professional examinations. Books and courses are available for the following specialties:

MRCP Part 1 and Part 2, MRCPCH Part 1 and Part 2, MRCOG, DRCOG, MRCGP, MRCPsych, DCH, FRCA, MRCS and PLAB.

For further details contact:

PasTest Ltd, Freepost, Knutsford, Cheshire, WA16 7BR

Tel: 01565 752000   Fax: 01565 650264
Email: enquiries@pastest.co.uk   **Web site: www. pastest.co.uk**

Typeset by Type Study, Scarborough, North Yorkshire
Printed by Alden Press, Oxfordshire

Contents

Contributors

Séamus Phillips is a Specialist Registrar in Otolaryngology on the South Thames ENT rotation. His specialist interests are Voice Pathology and Medical Engineering.

Lydia Badia is a Consultant ENT Surgeon at the Royal National Throat Nose and Ear Hospital, and an Honorary Senior Lecturer at the Institute of Laryngology and Otology, University College London. She specialises in Rhinology and Facial Plastic Surgery.

The authors and publishers would like to thank **Sudipta Banerjee MBChB MRCS** for allowing us to adapt her chapter 'Head, Neck, Endocrine and Paediatric', originally published in *MRCS System Modules: Essential Revision Notes*.

Acknowledgements

For their help with devising questions, the authors would like to thank:
Dr Anne Phillips, Specialist Registrar in Gastroenterology, West Midlands Rotation; ENT and Audiology Departments, Medway Maritime Hospital, Kent; ENT Senior House Officers, Medway Maritime Hospital, Kent.

For their help with images, the authors would like to thank:
Fiona Payne, Public Health Associate, London Public Health Training Programme; Dr Shivesh Kumar and Dr Shankar Ganesh, Senior House Officers in ENT, Medway Maritime Hospital, Kent.

Permissions

The following figures in this book have been reproduced with permission from: Becker, W., Nauman, H.H., Pfaltz, C.R., *Ear, Nose and Throat Diseases – A Pocket Reference*, 2nd edition. New York, NY: Thieme; 1994.

Fig. 2; Fig. 12; Fig. 15; Fig. 16; Fig. 17; Fig. 19; Fig. 20; Fig. 21; Fig. 22; Fig. 26; Fig. 31; Fig. 34; Fig. 35.

The following figures in this book have been reproduced with permission from: Snell, R., *Clinical Anatomy for Medical Students*, 6th edition. Philadelphia, PA: Lippincott, Williams and Wilkins; 2000.

Fig. 10; Fig. 13; Fig. 14; Fig. 18; Fig. 23; Fig. 24; Fig. 25; Fig. 27; Fig. 32; Fig. 33; Fig. 40; Fig. 41.

Introduction

Changes in training programmes are reducing the time junior doctors spend in various hospital departments before they move up to the specialist/GP registrar grade. It is important, therefore, that both knowledge and experience are acquired and consolidated during the short time spent in a specialty.

The Diploma in Otolaryngology – Head and Neck Surgery examination allows doctors to obtain a qualification as a result of ENT experience. The qualification is primarily designed for doctors who are not planning a career in ENT. However, it is also useful as a stepping stone to the FRCS examination for those moving on to specialist registrar training in ENT.

This book is aimed at candidates preparing for this examination, providing sample questions as well as summary revision notes in the most important areas. We also hope that it will prove useful for those studying for MRCS, MRCPCH and MRCGP examinations. Medical students these days find that their exposure to ENT is limited, yet they are examined in relative detail in this area – this book will also be of help to them.

Séamus Phillips
Lydia Badia

The DO-HNS Examination

STRUCTURE OF THE EXAM

The DO-HNS examination has two parts. Part 1 consists of a written paper with:

- **Multiple true/false questions** – these test basic knowledge in a wide range of ENT areas. They consist of a stem with associated statements, which are either true or false. There is no negative marking so it is best to guess even if you are not certain of the answer.
- **Extended matching questions** – these tend to concentrate more on clinical areas and case histories. Rather than being merely true or false, they have a wider range of possible answers, and as such you need more time to answer them fully.

The questions in Part 1 range across the whole syllabus, and it is better to cover quite a few areas in your revision rather than concentrate in depth on any one particular area. In particular, a wide range of basic science questions may be included, similar to those used in the MRCS examination, and if you are a not a surgeon but are taking the DO-HNS, you may benefit from reading MRCS revision material to expand your knowledge in this area. The paper is reasonably long, and you should make sure that you have the stamina to keep up concentration and performance for this time! You will also want to leave a little bit of time at the end for checking your answers and reconsidering those you are uncertain of.

Part 2 is the Objective Structured Clinical Examination (OSCE). Candidates rotate around a number of stations or bays, and each station has a question or clinical scenario:

- **Questions** require short written answers – it is important that these are legible and concise. The questions concentrate on common ENT problems and are usually based around photos, test results, anatomical diagrams or histological and pathological specimens. Examiners do not staff these stations, and candidates write answers down on separate answer sheets which they carry around with them.
- **Clinical scenarios** may include taking a history from an actor with a particular ENT problem, counselling a patient or relative, obtaining consent from a patient for a procedure or performing an ENT examination. An examiner is present and begins by giving the candidate a short instruction about what they need to do. In some cases the candidate will then have to read brief written instructions before commencing the scenario. The examiner will not provide further instructions but will merely observe the

candidate's performance. All equipment needed for examination is provided, although candidates may wish to bring their own otoscopes.

OSCEs are designed to make sure that all candidates are examined in the same areas in the same manner, and marking schemes are standardised so that all candidates are marked on the same criteria. So it is difficult to introduce bias. Because the written questions usually have at least one subsidiary question, it is taken into account that candidates who answer the first part of the question incorrectly, as such are misdirected in their answer to the second. In this case it is still possible to gain some marks for the second part, as long as the reasons for giving that answer follow logically from the first incorrect response.

Candidates move from one station to the next by a bell or other signal. A few rest stations are included in the 'circuit' where candidates have a chance to review answers that they may need to think more about. Candidates do not usually find that they are rushed in this examination, although the clinical stations do provide the pressure of an observer. Again, this examination requires stamina, as there is a constant need to change focus for the next station. In particular, if a clinical scenario station has gone badly in your opinion, do not let that affect your performance at the next station – think of each station change as a 'wiping of the slate' and a fresh start.

HINTS ON EXAM PREPARATION

Time should be set aside for revision, with study leave, if possible, close to the examination date. Revision timetables may help, as long as they do not set unrealistic goals! Speak to previous candidates and quiz them about the exam and their revision techniques. Attendance at a revision course may prove helpful in concentrating your mind on the syllabus without the distraction of daily clinical work.

Revision for Part 1 should cover a wide range of areas, including basic sciences as mentioned above. It should be done with close reference to the examination syllabus, and any areas that are not fully understood should be 'chased up' in textbooks until a deeper understanding is achieved. It may also be helpful to compile personalised revision notes in some form, which you can revisit closer to the examination. Practice sessions in answering MTFs and EMQs should be undertaken. It may also be helpful to devise one's own questions, perhaps with the aid of a colleague.

Revision for Part 2 differs, in that the range of areas covered is smaller. Reference to part 1 revision notes is helpful. However, it will also be useful to attend ENT clinics and practise examination skills under observation, so that basic ENT clinical examination is fluent and confident. This is particularly important if you are not currently in an ENT job. Feedback should be sought from seniors. Remember, it is not just the 'interesting patients' who should be examined – techniques can be practised on anyone, including colleagues! Books of 'picture tests' in ENT can also provide invaluable revision material.

Essential Revision Notes

CONTENTS

1   Basic Sciences

HEAD AND NECK ANATOMY

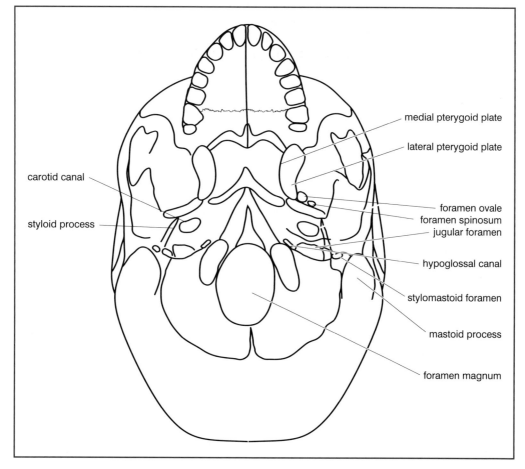

Fig. 1 The cranial fossa and nerves

Cranial nerves exit from various foramina in the skull (Table 1).

Foramen	Exiting structures
Optic canal	Optic nerve
	Ophthalmic artery
Superior orbital fissure	Ophthalmic vein
	Ophthalmic division of trigeminal nerve
	Oculomotor nerve
	Trochlear nerve
	Abducent nerve
Foramen rotundum	Maxillary division of trigeminal nerve
Foramen ovale	Mandibular division of trigeminal nerve
	Lesser petrosal branch of glossopharyngeal nerve
Foramen spinosum	Middle meningeal artery
Foramen lacerum	Internal carotid artery passes **across** foramen
	Greater petrosal branch of facial nerve
Internal auditory meatus	Vestibulocochlear nerve
	Facial nerve
Jugular foramen	Anterior compartment – glossopharyngeal nerve
	Middle compartment – vagus nerve, accessory nerve
Hypoglossal canal	Hypoglossal nerve
Foramen magnum	Spinal accessory nerve (entering)
Stylomastoid foramen	Temporal/zygomatic/buccal/mandibular/cervical/posterior auricular branches of facial nerve

Table 1 Foramina at the base of the skull and exiting structures

The external carotid artery has a number of branches, which supply various structures in the head and neck.

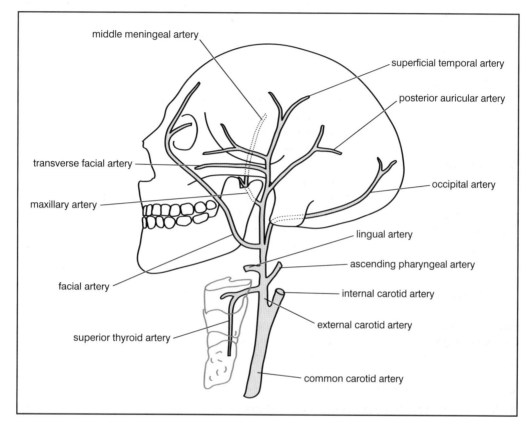

Fig. 2 The external carotid artery and its branches

INFLAMMATION

Inflammation is the response of the body to various types of injury, including:

◆ neoplastic
◆ infective
◆ traumatic
◆ autoimmune.

The resulting inflammation can be:

◆ acute – with a rapid onset and limited duration, or
◆ chronic – with a prolonged response and continuous repair taking place.

Acute inflammation

The classic components of the acute inflammatory response are:

◆ redness (rubor)
◆ swelling (tumor)
◆ heat (calor)
◆ pain (dolor)
◆ loss of function.

The response is caused by:

◆ local vasodilatation
◆ exudation of fluid and protein
◆ migration of leucocytes into the injured area.

The process is mediated by a number of chemical mediators:

◆ histamine
◆ cytokines
◆ nitric oxide
◆ protein components of plasma (complement system).

The complement system is a cascade of proteins, mutually activated in sequence, resulting in the lysing of microbes by the membrane attack complex (MAC). The most critical step is the activation of the C3 component:

◆ either by the **classical pathway** (triggered by an IgM or IgG antibody)
◆ or by the **alternative pathway** (triggered by exposure to the surface of the microbes).

Two other systems, the kinin system and the clotting system, also play a part in the acute inflammatory response.

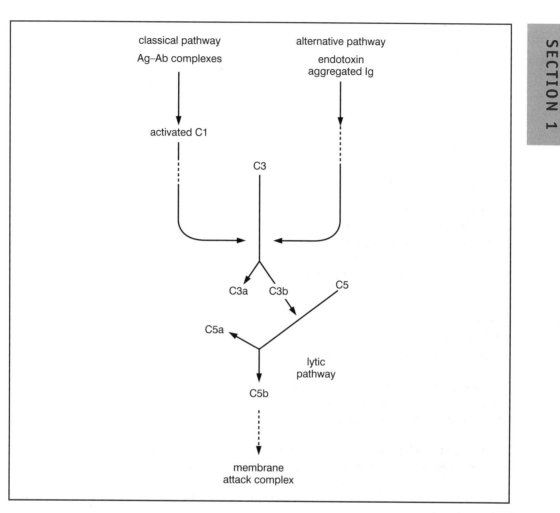

Fig. 3 The complement system

Chronic inflammation

Chronic inflammation is an ongoing but unresolved response to injury. Its characteristics are:

- proliferation of blood vessels and connective tissue
- migration of lymphocytes and macrophages
- fibrosis
- ongoing repair
- formation of granulomas.

Granulomas are focal areas of inflammation with a group of macrophages at the centre that transform into epithelial-like cells and are surrounded by a collar of lymphocytes and plasma cells. The epithelioid cells may fuse to form 'giant cells'. The inflammation may produce central caseating necrosis (classically in the case of tuberculosis (TB)) or may be non-caseating (most other chronic inflammations).

Response to inflammation

This depends on:

◆ the body's immune status
◆ the nature of the injuring agent
◆ the site of the injury.

After commencement of treatment, the response will also depend on choice of treatment and effective removal of the initial stimulus.

Infections may be classified as:

◆ conventional (infection in previously well individuals)
◆ conditional (infection in the presence of a predisposing factor)
◆ opportunistic (infection in an immunocompromised individual).

Most infections encountered in the ENT situation are conventional.

MICRO-ORGANISMS IN ENT INFECTION

Bacteria in ENT infection

The list below gives the classification of common bacteria encountered on a surgical ward, along with the situations in which some of them might be encountered in ENT.

Gram-positive

◆ Gram-positive cocci
  ● Aerobic
    − staphylococci (clusters)
    − *Staphylococcus aureus* – **wound infections, chronic suppurative otitis media (CSOM), acute sinusitis, furunculosis**
    − *S. epidermidis* – normal skin commensal
    − streptococci (chains/pairs) – **otitis externa**
    − α-haemolytic streptococcus
    − *Streptococcus pneumoniae* – **acute sinusitis, tonsillitis, acute suppurative otitis media (ASOM)**
    − *S. viridans*
    − β-haemolytic streptococcus – **tonsillitis**
    − Lancefield group A – *S. pyogenes* – **acute sinusitis**

- – Lancefield group B – *S. faecalis* – **dental infections**
- Anaerobic
  - – gut flora, *Enterococcus faecalis* – **tonsillitis, quinsy**
- ◆ Gram-positive bacilli
  - Aerobic
    - – *Corynebacterium diphtheriae*
  - Anaerobic
    - – *C. tetani*
    - – *C. difficile*
    - – *Actinomycetes israelii*

Gram-negative

- ◆ Gram-negative cocci
  - Aerobic
    - – *Neisseria meningitidis*
    - – *Moraxella catarrhalis* – **acute sinusitis, ASOM**
- ◆ Gram-negative bacilli
  - Aerobic
    - – *Pseudomonas aeruginosa* – **malignant otitis externa, tracheostomy infection**
    - – *Campylobacter*
    - – *Haemophilus influenzae* – **tonsillitis, epiglottitis, ASOM**
    - – *Legionella*
    - – *Escherichia coli* – **dental infections, tonsillitis, quinsy**
    - – *Proteus*
    - – *Mycobacterium tuberculosis* – **chronic ENT infections**
  - Anaerobic
    - – *Bacteroides fragilis*

Along with bacteria, fungi and viruses may also play a part in ENT disease.

Fungi in ENT infection

- ◆ *Aspergillus fumigatus* – this may cause **fungal sinusitis**, which is usually chronic but may be acute in immunocompromised individuals.
- ◆ *A. niger* – along with the other *Aspergillus* organisms, this may cause **fungal ear infections**.
- ◆ *Candida albicans* – this may cause **oral thrush**.

Viruses in ENT infection

Viral infection may be the precipitant cause for a bacterial tonsillitis. The following specific viruses are also encountered in ENT practice:

- ◆ Respiratory syncytial virus (RSV) – leads to chest infections, mainly in children in winter-time.

◆ Human immunodeficiency virus (HIV) – infects cells carrying the CD4 antigen, such as monocytes, macrophages and T-helper cells. More than half of patients may have head and neck manifestations such as otitis media, chronic rhinosinusitis, oropharyngeal Kaposi's sarcoma, lymphoma, herpes, or neck infections.

◆ Herpes – herpes zoster infection may lead to facial pain. In particular, if it affects the facial nerve, it may cause facial palsy. This is the Ramsay Hunt syndrome.

Antibiotics for ENT infections

The principles of antibiotic use in ENT are the same as in any branch of medicine. Effort should be made where possible to identify the causative organism before antibiotics are started. Some common ENT problems along with antibiotics indicated are given in Table 2. In all cases, erythromycin can be substituted for penicillin/amoxicillin if necessary.

Acute tonsillitis	Systemic penicillin – amoxicillin is avoided because of the risk of inducing a rash in cases of glandular fever
Quinsy/peritonsillar abscess	Systemic penicillin and metronidazole, with drainage
Acute otitis externa	Topical antibiotic drops with steroids
Malignant otitis externa	Systemic antibiotics, dependent on culture results
Acute otitis media	Systemic co-amoxiclav
Acute sinusitis	Systemic co-amoxiclav or second-generation cephalosporin
Chronic sinusitis	Broad-spectrum antibiotics initially
Epiglottitis	Chloramphenicol or third-generation cephalosporin
Cellulitis	Systemic flucloxacillin and penicillin
Wound infection	Dependent on wound culture
Post-tonsillectomy	Co-amoxiclav

Table 2 Common ENT infections and suggested antibiotics

ASSESSMENT FOR THEATRE

Fitness for ENT theatre depends on the following factors:

◆ the nature of the operation and anaesthetic that will be given
◆ the urgency of that operation
◆ the health of the patient preoperatively.

Preparation for theatre

Preparation for theatre may include the following:

History of the patient

This should include a history of the complaint leading to the need for the operation and its current status. Note should also be made of smoking and drinking history, drug history and family history.

Full examination

This should include auscultation of the heart and chest, and an ENT examination. The mouth should be examined as ENT operations often involve risk of damage to teeth – a loose tooth can be dislodged. Furthermore, pre-existing damage to teeth should be documented.

Special investigations

History and examination may reveal the need for an electrocardiogram (ECG) (in those over 60 years or with a history of cardiac problems), a chest X-ray (in those with clinical signs of chest disease) or an echocardiogram (in those with clinical signs of heart failure, or unexplained heart murmurs). Cross-match, group and save, full blood count, electrolytes, thyroid function, sickle cell status and/or clotting may be appropriate, depending on the nature of the operation and the patient's medical and drug history.

Thromboembolic and antibiotic prophylaxis

ENT operations rarely require antithrombotic prophylaxis, but in a patient with a history of thrombosis and likely immobility after an operation, mechanical and chemical prophylaxis may be indicated:

- Mechanical – thromboembolism-deterrent (TED) stockings, early mobilisation.
- Chemical – low molecular weight heparin is the most common agent, which should be discontinued 24 hours prior to administration or withdrawal of epidural anaesthesia/analgesia to prevent bleeding into the epidural space.

Antibiotic prophylaxis is rarely indicated in ENT surgery, but it may be necessary in patients with previous cardiac problems, patients who are immunocompromised, or operations where infection is likely to be present in or around the operation site.

Consent

It is important that patients being treated are fully aware as far as possible of what interventions are being proposed for their condition. To a certain extent, patients give 'implied' consent to basic actions such as history taking and examination by simply attending a medical facility. However, informed consent should be sought for any other intervention, as failure to do so may constitute an assault on the patient.

The procedure of obtaining informed consent may or may not involve the signing of a form, but in all cases the principles remain the same. An explanation of the following should be given:

◆ the details of the procedure
◆ the consequences if the procedure is not carried out
◆ the expected experiences during and after the procedure, such as pain levels
◆ the risks and potential side-effects, including a statistical likelihood if possible.

There should be an opportunity to ask questions.

Although it is often good practice to involve the family in any consent procedure, it is not mandatory. If an adult patient is not competent to give informed consent, the decision rests with the treating doctor to act in the patient's best interests. In these cases, all decisions must be carefully documented. Treatment may also be given in emergency situations without consent, as long as it is given in the patient's best interests. However, consent must be obtained as soon as the patient is capable of giving it.

For patients under 14 years of age consent should be obtained from the parents, although of course the child should not be left out of the conversation – a special consent form exists for the signature of the parents or appointed guardian (Form 3). For children aged 14 and 15, the doctor taking consent must make a judgement about whether the child is able to understand fully the procedure they are about to undergo, and all its implications and risks. The doctor should document this so-called 'Gillick competence' if the child is to sign the consent form.

A consent document is not legally binding; rather it acts as some degree of proof that a doctor has explained to a patient the nature of the procedure they are about to undergo and the risks of doing so. At any stage a patient may change their mind about proceeding.

There are certain situations where a doctor may treat without informed consent:

◆ A patient who is unconscious may be treated in their best interest, as long as no form of valid 'advance directive' exists to direct the medical personnel.
◆ Patients who are mentally incapable of making fully informed consent may be treated in their best interest – a special consent form exists for this purpose (Form 4), which is signed by the doctor only.

WOUNDS AND HEALING IN ENT

Wounds are created and repaired in the course of surgery, and it is essential to understand the process of wound healing, which consists of three phases:

◆ Acute inflammatory response – a clot is formed around the wound, with vasodilatation and influx of inflammatory cells, in particular neutrophils in the first 24 hours. Then the macrophages become more important, continuing the process of phagocytosis and secretion of cytokines (for example, transforming growth factor β (TGF-β), epidermal growth factor (EGF), platelet-derived growth factor (PDGF).

◆ Cell proliferation and deposition of extracellular matrix (proliferative phase) – fibroblasts secrete extracellular matrix and collagen; angiogenesis takes place, forming granulation tissue. There is wound contraction due to the action of myofibroblasts.

◆ Remodelling of the extracellular matrix (maturation phase) – lasts for many months and leads to a gradual increase in the strength of the wound, up to a maximum of 80%.

The commonest wounds in ENT surgery are of the face, an area that heals quickly given the right conditions. However, it is also an area about which the patient is highly sensitive with regard to slight asymmetry or changes in alignment. So, for the best result, care must be taken in the positioning of facial incisions to put the least possible tension on the healing wound. The skin has natural tension lines, and incisions placed on these lines tend to heal with a narrower and stronger scar, leading to more favourable results. In the face and neck they are most readily identified as the lines of wrinkling, and this fact can be used pre-operatively to mark the best possible position for an incision.

Delayed wound healing

Risk factors for delayed wound healing can be classified as follows:

◆ Local risk factors – infection, haematoma, mobility, foreign body, dirty wound, surgical technique, ischaemia.

◆ General risk factors – older age, cardiorespiratory disease, anaemia, obesity, diabetes mellitus, malnutrition, malignancy, steroids.

Poor healing may result in wound dehiscence, ie the partial or total disruption of layers of the operative wound.

Scars

All wounds form a scar in the process of repair. However, the healing response may become exaggerated. If excessive scar tissue is formed but is limited to the site of the original wound, a hypertrophic scar results. However, if the tissue extends beyond the boundaries of the original wound, a keloid scar results. Risk factors for hypertrophic and keloid scars include:

◆ young age
◆ black skin
◆ male sex
◆ genetic predisposition
◆ site – sternum, shoulders, head, neck

- wound tension
- delayed healing.

It is rare to find malignant change in a scar – if present, this is usually a squamous cell carcinoma, called 'Marjolin's ulcer'.

Drains in ENT

Head and neck surgery may result in wounds at risk of haematoma formation – if this is near the trachea, airway compromise may result, eg after thyroid surgery. To avoid this, drains may be placed in the area to minimise dead space. Drains in ENT are usually closed and often attached to a suction system, such as a Redivac drain. In the case of large abscesses, occasionally an open drainage system such as a Penrose or corrugated drain is left in situ after incision of the abscess.

HAEMATOLOGY

Haemostasis

Haemostasis is the cessation of bleeding, and involves a sequence of complex events:

- exposure of subendothelial tissue
- vasoconstriction
- adherence of platelets
- degranulation of platelets
- activation of the coagulation cascade
- platelet plug with fibrin support
- fibrinolysis and remodelling.

Platelets are a key factor – they bind to subendothelial collagen via von Willebrand's factor. They release their content(s), including fibrinogen and thromboxane A_2. The coagulation cascade is also a crucial factor, and it is shown in Fig. 4.

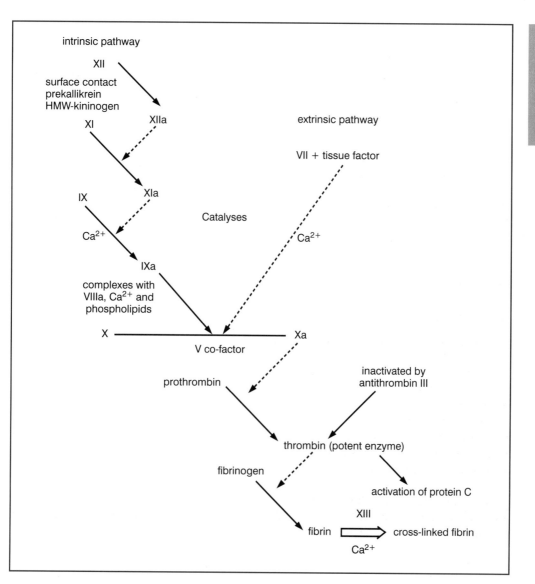

Fig. 4 The coagulation cascade

Fibrinolysis is carried out by plasmin, which is converted from inactive plasminogen by a number of factors, notably tissue plasminogen activator (tPA). Clotting time is measured by:

◆ activated partial thromboplastin time (APTT) – which measures the intrinsic as well as the common pathway
◆ prothrombin time (PT) – which measures the extrinsic as well as the common pathway
◆ thrombin time (TT) – which detects deficiencies of fibrinogen
◆ platelet count.

The way in which these times are altered gives a clue as to the underlying bleeding disorder, as shown in Table 3. Warfarin acts by blocking the synthesis of vitamin K-dependent factors and heparin activates antithrombin III, reducing fibrin formation – it is neutralised with protamine. Non-steroidal anti-inflammatory drugs (NSAIDs) affect the synthesis of thromboxane A_2 by platelets and thereby decrease their thrombotic action.

	PT	APTT	TT	Platelet count
Liver disease	Increased	Increased	Usually normal	Decreased
Warfarin	Increased	Usually normal	Normal	Normal
Heparin	Usually normal	Increased	Increased	Normal
Factor VII deficiency	Increased	Normal	Normal	Normal
Factor VIII deficiency	Normal	Increased	Normal	Normal
Factor XI deficiency	Normal	Increased	Normal	Normal
Disseminated intravascular coagulation	Increased	Increased	Increased	Decreased

Table 3 Changes in clotting times in various bleeding disorders

Haemophilia A is an X-linked deficiency in factor VIII, haemophilia B is also X-linked and is deficiency of factor XI – the two are clinically indistinguishable and are characterised by bleeding into soft tissue and joints after trauma. The commonest congenital bleeding disorder is von Willebrand's disease. There are also various congenital prothrombotic conditions – for example, protein C and S deficiencies, and antithrombin III deficiency.

Blood transfusion

Blood for transfusion comes from voluntary, healthy donors, and is known as 'whole blood'. However, it is usually split up into its constituent parts, namely:

♦ Red blood cell concentrates – plasma is removed, as it decays after a few days; this is the commonest transfused product but provides less volume replacement than whole blood; needs to be ABO-compatible.
♦ Platelet concentrates – can be used to treat thrombocytopenia or consumptive coagulopathy (eg disseminated intravascular coagulation (DIC)); needs to be ABO-compatible.

- Fresh frozen plasma (FFP) – contains all coagulation factors and can correct coagulopathies; needs to be ABO-compatible.
- Cryoprecipitate – produced by slow thawing of FFP; useful in the case of a fibrinogen deficiency, eg DIC.
- Factor concentrates – specific factor concentrates used to treat specific deficiencies.
- Albumin – only useful for diuretic-resistant oedema.

Red cells carry naturally occurring antigens, classified according to the ABO system. Other antigens may appear after sensitisation through transfusion or pregnancy. ABO incompatibility is the commonest cause of death due to transfusion – white cells or platelets may also produce a less severe transfusion reaction, due to the action of other antibodies. Other possible complications of blood transfusion are as follows:

- infection, eg HIV, hepatitis, human T-lymphotrophic virus (HTLV)
- fluid/iron overload
- hypothermia
- hyperkalaemia
- hypocalcaemia
- metabolic acidosis
- acute respiratory distress syndrome (ARDS)
- DIC.

ANALGESIA

Physiology of pain

Pain is defined as an unpleasant sensory and emotional experience associated with actual or potential tissue damage. There are four stages:

1 **Transduction** – tissue damage results in the release of arachidonic acid metabolites such as leukotrienes, prostaglandins and thromboxane A_2. These act at free nerve endings.
2 **Transmission** – free nerve ending stimulation transmits pain along A and C fibres.
3 **Modulation** – natural and synthetic opioids may act centrally or in the spinal column via opioid receptors to modulate the pain experience. Mechanical stimulation (eg rubbing) may also inhibit pain.
4 **Perception** – this occurs in the thalamus and sensory cortex.

Pain control

Pain is managed best by anticipating it, rather than by waiting for it to manifest itself. It often requires more than one analgesic agent. Options for analgesia are as follows:

- Opioids – these may be given orally, intravenously, intramuscularly or topically. They act at opioid receptors, and have many side-effects, such as constipation, nausea, respiratory depression and addiction. They may be given in the form of a patient-controlled system, which allows the patient to anticipate their own analgesic needs.
- Local anaesthetics – local infiltration into the wound, a regional block or an epidural block may produce profound analgesia but side-effects such as hypotension and respiratory depression should be monitored.
- NSAIDs – these have anti-inflammatory, analgesic and antipyretic properties; side-effects include gastric damage, bronchospasm and gout.

ANAESTHESIA FOR ENT

Anaesthesia is defined as the rendering of part or all of the body insensitive to pain or noxious stimuli. Anaesthesia for ENT procedures presents challenges that are slightly different in comparison with anaesthesia for other procedures.

General anaesthesia

ENT procedures often involve relatively minor procedures on relatively fit patients. However, major operations on head and neck cancers involve substantial risk to the airway in patients who smoke on a regular basis and have other anaesthetic risk factors. Other airway operations on patients with obstructive apnoea will require careful anaesthetic monitoring before, during and after the procedure. Insertion of a tracheostomy or correction of airway stenosis involves careful co-ordination with the anaesthetist to ensure a safe airway throughout the procedure. General anaesthesia induces narcosis, analgesia and muscle relaxation.

General anaesthesia – usual sequence

- Premedication/sedation
- Induction of anaesthesia
- Muscle relaxation
- Maintenance of anaesthesia
- Reversal of anaesthesia and recovery

Premedication

Premedication is not compulsory, but it may be necessary to lessen anxiety, dry secretions, prevent anaesthetic-related emesis or increase vagal tone. Common agents for pre-medication are:

- benzodiazepines, eg midazolam
- opioids, eg morphine

◆ anticholinergics, eg glycopyrrolate
◆ antacids, eg cimetidine.

Operations on the nasal passages often require vasoconstriction to decrease mucosal swelling, and this is achieved by application of an intranasal solution preoperatively. A common choice is Moffett's solution (a mixture of cocaine, adrenaline, sodium bicarbonate and saline).

Induction of anaesthesia

Anaesthesia can be induced by inhalational or intravenous (iv) agents. Propofol is a commonly used iv agent (thiopental sensitises the pharynx and cannot be used with laryngeal airways). Children may require inhalation of a gas such as halothane. These agents act quickly to lower the level of consciousness to one conducive to the operation. Complications of induction agents include laryngeal spasm that may exacerbate airway problems.

Muscle relaxation

Paralysis is sometimes employed in ENT procedures. **Depolarising muscle relaxants**, such as suxamethonium, act quickly on acetylcholine receptors to cause muscle fasciculation and then relaxation. Suxamethonium has a short half-life, but it cannot be used in patients with a history of bronchospasm, myasthenia gravis or malignant hyperpyrexia.

Non-depolarising agents such as atracurium have a slower onset but last longer. They can be reversed by means of neostigmine. Patients with myasthenia gravis are more sensitive to non-depolarising agents than other patients. For ENT procedures in patients with difficult airways, muscle relaxation should be used with caution as it may leave the patient apnoeic and needing ventilation, which may then be difficult to administer.

Maintenance of anaesthesia

This is usually achieved by inhalational agents:

◆ enflurane
◆ isoflurane
◆ sevoflurane.

Nitrous oxide is only a weak anaesthetic but potentiates the effects of other anaesthetics. Hence it is often used in conjunction with them. However, it diffuses rapidly into any air-containing space and so increases the pressure in the middle ear. This can lead to problems with middle-ear grafts, as their position may be altered by this increase in pressure.

Surgery that involves a risk of bleeding in the laryngeal or tracheal area presents a particular challenge for the anaesthetist, as it can precipitate airway compromise. Laser use in the airway carries a risk of fire, and precautions should be taken, such as the use of a metallic tracheal tube and filling of the cuff with saline.

Local anaesthesia

◆ This involves temporary blockage of transmission of nerve impulses by altering the permeability of the membranes of nerve cells.
◆ It may be used alone or in combination with a general anaesthetic to increase analgesia.
◆ Acidic solutions are used – which are prompted to work by the alkalinity of the surrounding tissue. So, in infected, acidic conditions they may not be effective.

Local anaesthetic may be administered in a number of different ways:

◆ topical, eg application of Moffett's solution to the nose for intranasal procedures
◆ direct infiltration, eg lidocaine for excision of superficial lesions or suturing
◆ nerve block, eg the superior laryngeal nerve (applying lidocaine to the pyriform fossae)

Epidural/spinal anaesthetics are not used for ENT procedures.

Complications

◆ Toxicity – inadvertent iv administration or over-rapid absorption may lead to perioral effects, which progress to drowsiness, seizures, coma and collapse; all local anaesthetics have maximum doses dependent on weight – this maximum may be increased by the use of agents such as adrenaline, which slow absorption and prolong period of action.
◆ Allergic reaction – this usually causes an immediate reaction and may lead to bronchospasm, laryngeal oedema or cardiovascular collapse. Adrenaline and iv fluids should be given, and antihistamines and bronchodilators may be necessary.

OPERATING EQUIPMENT FOR ENT SURGERY

As in all branches of surgery, ENT has many specialised operating tools. These can be classified as follows:

◆ equipment used to carry out procedures in the outpatient department, eg wax hooks, microsuction, nasal specula, cautery sticks
◆ equipment used to carry out particular operations, eg ear micro-instruments, tonsil retractors, laryngoscopes, oesophagoscopes
◆ airway adjuncts, eg tracheostomy tubes, stents
◆ aids to visualisation, eg microscopes, nasoendoscopes, functional endoscopic sinus surgery (FESS) instruments.

Laser

Lasers are being used increasingly in ENT surgery. Laser stands for **L**ight **A**mplification by **S**timulated **E**mission of **R**adiation, and provides a way of directing energy to a very specific point. This energy can be focused using lenses, and its effects on surrounding tissue vary according to the type of laser used, the duration of action and the density of the beam.

Uses of laser in ENT surgery

- Ear – fine surgery around ossicles and stapedectomy, welding of grafts.
- Nose – cautery, dacryocystorhinostomy, management of hereditary haemorrhagic telangiectasia (HHT).
- Throat – excision of benign lesions, debulking of tumours.

IMAGING/RADIOLOGY

ENT uses all modes of imaging to aid diagnosis and treatment.

Plain X-rays

These may be used in the case of sinus disease but have now been superseded by computed tomography (CT) scans. Lateral neck X-rays are often taken in cases of suspected foreign bodies in the throat. However, there is often very little useful information to be gained as foreign bodies may not be radio-opaque and may be confused with normal structures in the throat.

Computed tomography

CT scans provide information about bony structures and soft tissues in the head and neck area. Sinus disease is well visualised, and iodine contrast provides further information about abnormal blood flow in lymph node enlargement and neoplasia. Dense bone in the skull base area is not well visualised, but the temporal bone is well seen.

Magnetic resonance imaging (MRI)

MRI performs well in imaging soft tissue. It works by aligning protons in living tissue in magnetic fields, which then relax when the field is turned off and produce radio waves that can be received and analysed. The signal is composed of two components, T1 and T2.

- T1 component relates to the time taken for spinning protons to return to their normal position – T1-weighted images provide high anatomical definition, including the soft tissues.
- T2 is related to excited protons moving out of phase with each other – T2 images show up abnormal tissue better, such as inflamed and neoplastic tissue.
- Short tau inversion recovery (STIR)-weighted images are similar to T2 but with fat signal suppression, which can provide clearer information about the outline of tumours.
- Gadolinium is a commonly used contrast agent and, like iodine, shows up areas of increased vascularity.

Ultrasound

Ultrasound is an effective, quick and safe method of imaging soft-tissue swellings in the head and neck area. It can be used in conjunction with fine-needle aspiration to provide further information. It is, however, very operator-dependent.

Contrast studies

Barium swallows are commonly done for the assessment of swallowing problems, pharyngeal webs and pharyngeal pouches. If aspiration, perforation or leakage is a risk, water-soluble contrast can be used.

IMMUNOLOGY

Physiology of the immune system

Stimulation of the immune system by exposure to pathogens leads to increased resistance to that pathogen in the future. The components of the immune system can be classified as:

◆ **non-specific defences**, such as skin, complement system and neutrophils
◆ **specific defences**, such as lymphocytes, which are triggered by exposure to antigens.

The sequence of events in the immune response is as follows :

1 Antigens are 'presented' by any cell using the class I major histocompatibility complex (MHC) molecule (Table 4) or by dendritic cells and macrophages, which use the class II MHC molecule.
2 A peptide fragment of the antigen is then combined with the relevant MHC molecule and expressed on the cell surface.
3 Class I MHC molecules are recognised by CD8+ T lymphocytes (cytotoxic T cells) which kill cells infected with the pathogen. Class II molecules are recognised by CD4+ T-helper cells, which produce soluble immune system mediators such as interferons and interleukins.
4 These substances then stimulate various specific aspects of the immune system. B lymphocytes are stimulated as a result and differentiate into plasma cells. These cells secrete immunoglobulins, helped by T-helper cells.

MHC type	Found in	Recognised by	Effect
Class I	Every cell	CD8+ T-cytotoxic cell	Kills infected cells
Class II	Macrophages/dendritic cells	CD4+ T-helper cell	Production of immune system mediators

Table 4 Major histocompatibility complex class I and II

Structure of immunoglobulins

Immunoglobulins are antibodies that have the structure shown in Fig. 5. They are made up of a constant and a variable region, or can also be thought of as a light and heavy chain, or an Fab (antigen-binding) fragment and an Fc (complement) fragment. The binding of antibodies to antigen leads to lysis of bacteria, initiation of the classical complement pathway and killing of the infected cell, among other effects.

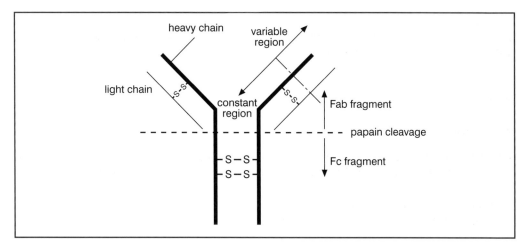

Fig. 5 Antibody structure

Classification of immune responses

The immune system may respond inappropriately to activation by antigens in a **hypersensitivity reaction**. These responses have been classified by Gell and Coombs as shown in the box.

- **Type I (anaphylactic or immediate)** – exposure leads to IgE formation. This binds to mast cells and basophils, leading to release of mediators on subsequent exposure. Hay fever, anaphylactic reaction and allergic rhinitis are examples. Sodium cromoglycate and steroids may act to inhibit mediator release by stabilising lysosomal membranes.
- **Type II (cytotoxic)** – this is mediated by antibodies against antigens, and results in the activation of cells themselves or of complement, leading to cell damage. Examples are graft rejection and transfusion reaction.
- **Type III (immune complex-mediated)** – immune complexes of antigen with antibody lead to complement activation and tissue damage. An example is systemic lupus erythematosus (SLE).
- **Type IV (cell-mediated/delayed)** – this reaction is mediated by sensitised T lymphocytes, leading to T-cell activation and recruitment of macrophages, resulting in damage. TB and transplant rejection are examples.
- **Type V (stimulatory)** – antireceptor antibodies stimulate cell function. Examples are Graves' disease and myasthenia gravis.

PHYSIOLOGY FOR ENT

Cardiac physiology

In any surgical specialty, a basic knowledge of physiology is important. In particular, cardiovascular and respiratory function may be relevant to a patient's pre-, peri- and post-operative management.

Heart muscle is specialised to perform involuntary pulsatile contraction. Its structure is similar to skeletal muscle, ie it is made up of sarcomeres, which, in turn, are made up of thick (myosin) and thin (actin) filaments. The force that each sarcomere can exert partly depends on the initial length of that sarcomere. In other words, when the sarcomere is very short, or very long, less force is exerted. There exists an optimal length of sarcomere at which maximum force is exerted on contraction. **Starling's curve** (Fig. 6) is based on this characteristic.

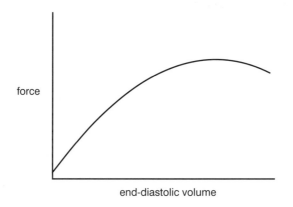

Fig. 6 Starling's curve

Up to a point, therefore, increasing the blood volume in the heart can increase the force of contraction of the heart. Cardiac output and stroke volume also vary in the same way with end-diastolic volume. Another factor that increases contractility of the heart is the concentration of calcium ions in the cells – more intracellular calcium results in a greater force of contraction.

Cardiac cells transmit a contraction impulse between each other and so contract in a synchronised fashion. A wave of depolarisation passes through the heart by this means. Contraction is initiated by the sino-atrial and atrioventricular nodes as well as the Purkinje fibres in the ventricles. All these cells have their own intrinsic rate of impulse generation (self-excitation). The sinoatrial node fires the fastest, at a rate of around 100 beats per minute (bpm). The atrioventricular node is next, and the Purkinje fibres fire at 40 bpm. If the sinoatrial node fails to fire, the cells with the next highest rate of firing will take over.

Vagal activity slows the intrinsic firing rate and sympathetic hormones and sympathetic innervation increase it. Sympathetic nerve fibres (C8–T5) cause noradrenaline release at nerve endings, acting on cardiac β receptors, increasing heart rate and force. Parasympathetic fibres (via the vagus nerve) cause acetylcholine release, which acts on muscarinic receptors and causes a slowing of the heart rate.

Regulation of stroke volume takes place due to the following factors:

◆ Preload – Starling's Law implies that the initial fibre stretch of the cardiac muscle will influence stroke volume. This in turn depends on filling time of the atria and how much compliance (stretchability) is present.
◆ Contractility – this is increased by preload, the presence of hormones such as adrenaline, thyroxine and glucagons, and by certain drugs. It is decreased by hypoxia, acidosis and alkalosis, electrolyte imbalance, and of course by drugs.
◆ Afterload – this is the tension of the ventricular walls required to eject the blood into the systemic circulation. Aortic stenosis and increased systemic vascular resistance increase afterload and vasodilators decrease it.

Transport of oxygen

◆ Oxygen is mostly transported bound to haemoglobin.
◆ Haemoglobin contains four O_2-binding haem molecules.
◆ A small amount of O_2 is also transported dissolved in plasma
◆ The oxygen dissociation curve (Fig. 7) determines the relation between O_2 saturation and PaO_2.

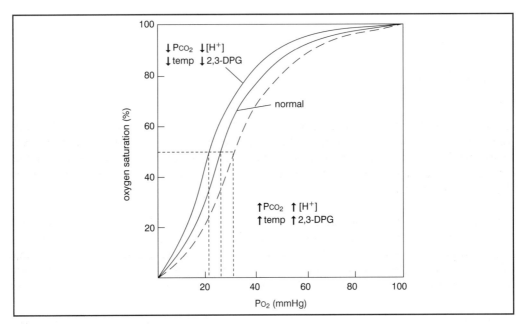

Fig. 7 Oxygen dissociation curve

Factors shifting curve to the left (increased affinity for O_2):

◆ decreased $PaCO_2$
◆ decreased $[H^+]$ (Bohr effect)
◆ decreased 2,3-DPG
◆ decreased temperature
◆ HbF, carboxyhaemoglobin.

The opposite will shift the curve to the right.

Transport of carbon dioxide

CO_2 is transported in three ways:

◆ dissolved as CO_2 in plasma
◆ reacts with amines in deoxyhaemoglobin to form carboxyhaemoglobin
◆ reacts with H_2O to form H^+ and HCO_3^-, transported as sodium bicarbonate.

Deoxyhaemoglobin is a weaker acid than oxyhaemoglobin and can carry more CO_2 (Haldane's effect).

Control of respiration

Respiration is controlled by a number of feedback loops based on chemo-, baro- and mechanoreceptors, as well as voluntary control. These mechanisms as shown in Fig. 8.

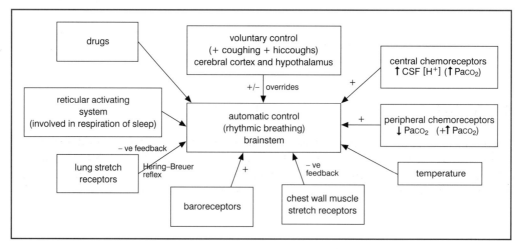

Fig. 8 Control of respiration. Hering–Breuer reflex = negative feedback from lung stretch receptors as the lung inflates

AIDS TO VENTILATION

If a patient's ventilation is inadequate, intubation of some kind may be necessary. Endotracheal intubation is indicated in the following cases:

◆ Glasgow Coma Scale (GCS) score < 8
◆ impaired gag reflex
◆ to prevent a rise in intracranial pressure (ICP)
◆ to enable suction of secretions
◆ severe hypoxia or metabolic acidosis
◆ risk of upper airway obstruction.

A cuff prevents aspiration, but may cause stenosis and tracheomalacia if the pressure is too high. When endotracheal intubation is not possible, a surgical airway may be necessary. In an emergency, **surgical cricothyroidotomy** is performed, ie an incision made in the cricothyroid membrane and a cuffed tube is inserted. In a more controlled situation, there are other options:

◆ Surgical tracheostomy – an incision is made through the second and third tracheal rings. It is indicated in the following situations:
  ● when weaning off an endotracheal (ET) tube
  ● to enable suction of secretions
  ● chronic ventilation
  ● to facilitate oral care.
◆ Percutaneous tracheostomy – this technique involves progressive dilation of a puncture hole in the trachea, which does not require transfer to theatre, and may be performed by doctors in an intensive care unit (ICU).
◆ Mini-tracheostomy – a small tracheostomy tube is inserted in the cricothyroid membrane to enable suctioning of secretions, but it is not suitable as a definitive airway as it is not cuffed.

CLINICAL GOVERNANCE AND AUDIT

The concept of clinical governance is a relatively new one. It complements the increased autonomy of financial governance that has been introduced in the British health system, and **gives clinicians responsibility for monitoring their own group and individual performance and improving that performance continuously**. Various aspects of clinical governance include:

◆ audit
◆ evidence-based medicine (EBM)
◆ continuing education
◆ teaching
◆ research
◆ risk management.

Audit

For surgeons in training, audit is one of the commonest methods by which they will be involved in clinical governance. Audit is the process by which clinical staff collectively review, evaluate and improve their practice with the aim of improving standards. From this definition follows the structure of the audit cycle (Fig. 9).

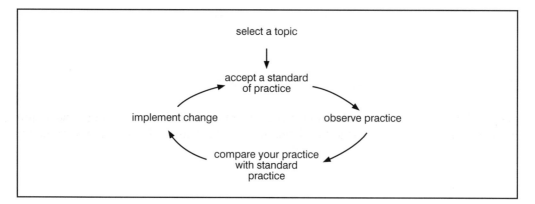

Fig. 9 Audit cycle

Evidence-based medicine

EBM is the practice of basing medical decisions on research. It involves:

- formulating the clinical question to be answered
- gathering evidence on this question
- assessing the quality and applicability of the evidence available
- arriving at a conclusion about the appropriate decision for the individual case being considered.

This process includes a critical appraisal of the literature involved. Double-blind randomised controlled trials represent the best quality evidence, but these may not always exist or even be possible. Studies may be subject to bias not mentioned in the publication, for example:

- Publication bias – negative findings are less likely to be published.
- Response bias – those not responding may be at the extreme ends of the range of subjects studied.
- Analysis bias – randomised controlled trials should be analysed on an intention-to-treat basis, not according to what treatment the patient finally ended up receiving: this is because, in real life, patients are free to change treatments, and it is the initial management strategy that is being assessed.

2 Audiology

CLINICAL ASSESSMENT OF HEARING

Simple clinical assessments of hearing may give a clue about the nature of the underlying problem. Although more sophisticated hearing tests such as audiograms are in common use, they are not always easily accessible.

Voice testing

It is of course difficult to standardise voice testing of hearing. The general procedure for free-field voice testing is as follows:

1   Test each ear separately with a whispered voice, conversational voice and a loud voice at 60 cm.
2   Repeat at 15 cm.
3   Mask the contralateral ear.
4   Ask the patient to repeat the two-word phrases uttered by the examiner.

The most difficult test is performed first (whispered voice at 60 cm, then at 15 cm) and then the tests become easier until at least 50% of the words are repeated correctly. Masking is most easily performed by gently rubbing the tragus of the contralateral ear with the index finger of one hand.

Tuning fork tests

These tests provide a guide to the presence of hearing loss and suggest the nature of that loss. They involve the use of a tuning fork, ideally at 512 Hz or 256 Hz, with a footplate to enable good contact with the skull.

- **Rinne's test** involves the comparison of bone and air conduction on each side separately, ideally with masking of the other side. A positive response is when air conduction is perceived as louder than bone conduction and indicates no hearing loss or a sensorineural loss. A negative response indicates a conductive hearing loss.
- **Weber's test** involves placing the tuning fork in a central position in contact with the skull and asking which ear the sound localises to. Localisation to one side indicates a

conductive hearing loss on that side or, alternatively, a sensorineural loss on the other side. This test can detect a difference of 10 dB.

- **Stenger's test** is used to differentiate feigned from genuine hearing loss. It is based on the observation that if two identical tones are presented to either ear, the individual will only hear the louder one. Two tuning forks of the same frequency are used:
  - Ask the individual to close their eyes.
  - Present the first tuning fork 15 cm from the good ear – they will hear it.
  - Place the second 5 cm from the bad ear – they will deny hearing it.
  - With this still in place, re-present the first tuning fork 15 cm from the good ear.
  - If the hearing loss is genuine, the individual will notice the first tuning fork – if not, they will only hear the second at the 'bad' ear and will say they do not hear anything.

Audiograms

- Pure tone audiogram (PTA) involves the measurement of the minimum amplitude that can be heard at a certain frequency.
- Measurements are given in decibels, the measure of sound intensity.
- The normal ear hears certain frequencies better than others and so an unadjusted graph of frequency against decibel thresholds would not be flat. The hearing level scale (dB HL) adjusts the threshold so that 0 dB represents the normal hearing level, whatever the frequency.
- Air conduction is assessed by pure tones presented via headphones, with masking of the contralateral ear via the headphones.
- A skull vibrator assesses bone conduction, with masking by an ear insert.
- Tones are presented at various frequencies from 250 Hz to 8000 Hz, with amplitude reduced in 10-dB steps until no tones are heard and then increased in 5-dB steps until half the tones are heard.

It is important to note that treatment of a middle ear ossicular discontinuity causes an artificial increase in the bone conduction thresholds – this is known as the **Carhart effect**, and a loss of bone conduction at 2000 Hz due to ossicular pathology (eg otosclerosis) is known as a **Carhart notch**.

Assessment of vestibular function

The body maintains balance by using information received from the vestibular system, the eyes and the muscles. Two reflexes are used to elicit information about the balance system.

Vestibulo-ocular reflex

Eye movements must be assessed first before the vestibulo-ocular reflex can be relied upon to give information about the vestibular system itself; normal saccades (quick movement from one side to the other) and pursuit (following a pendulum) should be present.

Stimulation of the vestibular system should induce **nystagmus**, which is an involuntary rhythmic oscillation of the eyes.

◆ True vestibular nystagmus consists of a slow movement of the eyes in one direction followed by a quick corrective movement in the opposite direction.
◆ The slow movement is generated by signals from the vestibule.
◆ The quick movement is of central origin.
◆ The nystagmus will be worst when looking in the direction of the fast component.
◆ The direction of the nystagmus is named after the direction of the fast component.

Tests designed to stimulate the vestibular system may be performed – the resulting nystagmus is a signal that that system is working correctly.

◆ **Rotational tests** stimulate both vestibules simultaneously by rotating the subject.
◆ **Caloric tests**, involving infusion of cold water at 30 °C, generate a convection current in the endolymph on that side. This will elicit a vestibular response in the form of nystagmus if the vestibule is functioning correctly. The test is also performed with hot water at 44 °C. Cold water leads to nystagmus with the fast phase towards the opposite side. The mnemonic COWS (cold-opposite, warm-same) can be used to remember the expected response to the test. Lack of response may indicate a peripheral vestibular failure on one side.

Vestibulospinal reflex

Various tests use this reflex to provide information about the vestibular system.

◆ **Romberg's test** – the patient stands still with arms by the sides and eyes closed. If there is an uncompensated vestibular lesion on one side, the patient will show a tendency to fall to that side.
◆ **Unterberger's test** – the patient marches on the spot with arms outstretched and eyes closed for 30 seconds. An abnormal response is a rotation of at least 30° or a forwards or backwards movement of at least 1 m.

EVOKED RESPONSE AUDIOMETRY

This is the measurement of automatic auditory system responses to sound and does not require the patient to be conscious.

Electrocochleography (EcochG)

◆ Reference electrode is placed on the mastoid.
◆ Active electrode stimulates the promontory through the tympanic membrane.
◆ Test signal is transmitted via earphones; response is measured.
◆ EcochG can be used to test thresholds accurately in very young children and also for intraoperative monitoring of hearing.

Brainstem electrical response audiometry (BERA)

- Electrodes are placed over the mastoid, forehead and vertex.
- The patient is awake but must lie still.
- Stimulate via headphones.
- The resulting waves are characterised as levels I–V, depending on their position in the auditory neural pathway.
- Latency (time delay) is analysed.
- BERA can be used to investigate acoustic neuroma and brainstem lesions.

Cortical response audiometry

- Vertex potential is a delayed cortical response to sound and is associated with the perception of hearing.
- It is measured with vertex electrodes.
- Patient must be still and co-operative.

Otoacoustic emissions (OAEs)

The outer hair cells have a motor function, ie they dampen vibrations on either side of the target frequency. OAEs are vibrations of the outer hair cells that are a result of the ear's capacity to 'fine tune' its frequency sensitivity depending on the sound being detected.

- An ear probe stimulates the cells by means of click sounds.
- This stimulation produces emissions from the outer hair cells, which are detected by the microphone included in the probe apparatus.
- OAEs are used for screening neonates for hearing function.

HEARING AIDS

Components of hearing aids

- Microphone
- Amplifier
- Sound transmitter
- Power source

- Hearing aids process external sounds and present them to the inner ear in a way that can be interpreted by the brain.
- Signals can be processed by analogue or digital means.
- Analogue aids can reduce sounds that are above a certain level to avoid uncomfortable peaks.
- Digital processing can adjust the signal to selectively increase certain frequencies or to minimise background noise.

Types of hearing aid

◆ Postaural aids – these are worn behind the ear and contain an induction coil that can be used to pick up sound from televisions and in theatres.
◆ In-the-ear aids – these are smaller and more expensive than behind-the-ear aids, and they are prone to auditory feedback (reamplification of generated sound to produce a whistling noise).
◆ Body-worn aids – these are bigger and so can amplify sounds better but are cumbersome.
◆ Bone conduction aids – sounds are transmitted to a vibrator strapped to the skull.
◆ Osseo-integrated aids – these attach permanently to the skull and are vibrated, either directly or by induction, by an external transmitter. Sounds are then transmitted via bone conduction; these are also known as bone-anchored hearing aids (BAHA).
◆ Implantable middle ear aids – an external transmitter vibrates a receiver attached directly to the incus.
◆ Cochlear implants – an array is implanted directly into the cochlea, which is thought to stimulate the auditory nerve directly. Sounds are picked up behind the ear and processed using various speech-coding strategies, and then the array is stimulated by induction.

Careful selection of those undergoing cochlear implantation is necessary. Neural plasticity is a major factor:

◆ if the auditory pathway is not exposed to sounds by the age of 8 months, the ability to listen is lost
◆ if speech is not heard by the age of 3 years, speech articulation is not possible.

A patient is classed as post-lingually deaf if speech is acquired before deafness, and cochlear implantation is possible. In prelingually deaf children, implantation must be done before listening ability is lost. Candidacy for implantation also depends on auditory assessment, a disease-free ear, radiological examination (including an MRI scan) and a psychological assessment to ensure that the patient's expectations are realistic.

Presbycusis

Various changes occur with age in the hearing mechanism:

◆ reduction in the number of inner and outer hair cells
◆ cell death due to arterial disease
◆ degeneration of central pathways.

This leads to sensorineural loss, which begins at high frequencies and causes difficulty in discrimination in the presence of background noise. One-fifth of those in their seventh decade have at least a moderate hearing impairment.

Management

- Hearing aids – care must be taken to fit a suitable aid, as non-compliance is high
- Accessory aids, eg induction coils
- Rehabilitation, eg lip-reading training

TINNITUS

- Tinnitus is the sensation of sound not resulting from external stimuli.
- Up to 8% of the population may present to the medical profession complaining of it.
- A minority of these find that it affects their quality of life.
- The majority of sufferers also have some degree of hearing loss.
- Almost all ear diseases can be associated with the development of tinnitus, as well as many pathologies of the cardiovascular or neurological systems.
- Objective tinnitus may be detected by others and may result from palatal myoclonus or vascular malformations, amongst other things.
- A full history should be taken, along with an examination of the auditory and vestibular systems, including an audiogram.
- MRI may be necessary in the case of unilateral tinnitus as acoustic neuromas may present in this way.
- Pulsatile tinnitus may require angiography or other imaging investigation to rule out vascular causes.

There are many theories of the cause of tinnitus, all based around the fact that an electrical potential is being generated in the auditory pathway by damaged nerves or faulty central processing. After management of any underlying cause, treatment is directed at habituating the patient to the tinnitus by means of hearing aids and white-noise generators, as well as counselling. Self-help advice and reassurance may be extremely helpful.

3 Otology

EMBRYOLOGICAL ORIGIN OF EAR STRUCTURES

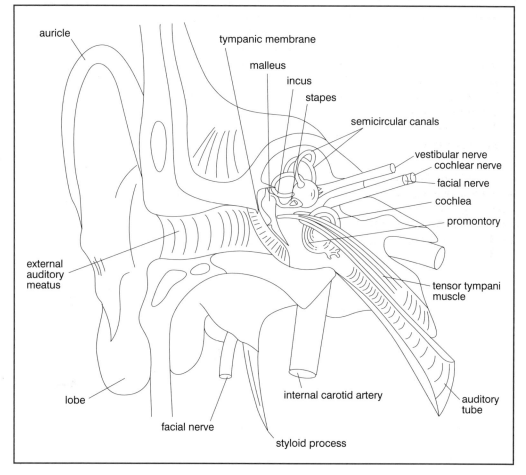

Fig. 10 Anatomy of the ear

Structure	Embryological origin
Malleus, incus, stapedius	1st arch
Stapes, tensor tympani	2nd arch
Middle ear	1st pharyngeal pouch

Table 5 Embryological origin of the structures of the ear

EXTERNAL EAR

Anatomy

The external ear has a number of constituent parts (Fig. 11):

◆ helix
◆ antihelix
◆ tragus
◆ antitragus
◆ lobe.

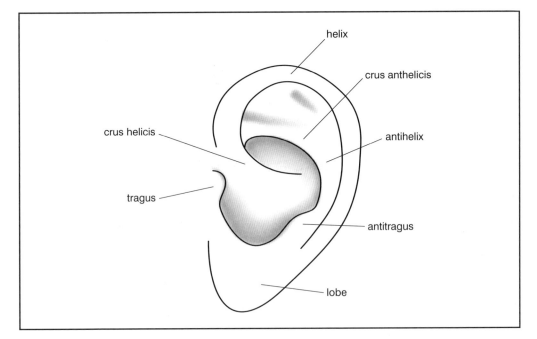

Fig. 11 The external ear

The nerve supply of the external ear is as follows:

- upper lateral surface – auriculotemporal nerve from mandibular nerve
- lower lateral surface and medial surface – greater auricular nerve from C3
- skin posterior to ear – lesser occipital nerve from C2/C3.

Ear trauma

Trauma to the ear is a frequent occurrence, and severe cases may require the attention of a plastic surgeon. However, the commonest complaints can be dealt with by ENT surgeons without a general anaesthetic:

- Lacerations not involving the main body of the ear cartilage can be sewn with nylon sutures in the same way as other lacerations.
- Bites to the ear must be left open and treated with antibiotics.
- Pinna haematomas should be drained via an incision at the back of the ear, with the insertion of a small drain if necessary and the suturing of a dental roll on either side of the ear cartilage, with pressure applied with a head bandage.
- Failure to adequately drain blood accumulating in the subperichondrial space may lead to death of the underlying cartilage and a consequent deformation of the pinna, commonly known as a 'cauliflower ear'.

Protruding ears

Protruding ears, or 'bat ears':

- These are caused by the absence of the antihelical fold in the auricular cartilage.
- Treatment involves surgical exposure of the lateral aspect of the cartilage behind the pinna and scoring it to produce a rounded fold.

EAR CANAL AND TYMPANIC MEMBRANE

Anatomy

The ear canal is lined by stratified squamous epithelium and is made up of:

- outer one third – cartilage
- inner two-thirds – temporal bone.

Sensory supply to the ear canal and external tympanic membrane:

- anterior – auriculotemporal nerve
- superior – facial nerve
- posterior – lesser occipital nerve
- inferior – vagus nerve.

The relevant branch of the vagus is known as Alderman's nerve, which supplies the inferior part of the tympanic membrane as well as part of the canal. This gives rise to the phenomenon that patients may cough while having their ears suctioned.

The medial end of the canal is formed by the tympanic membrane and the anatomy is shown in Fig. 12. The medial surface of the tympanic membrane is the lateral limit of the middle ear. It is lined with pseudostratified columnar epithelium anteriorly and flat or cuboidal epithelium posteriorly. The pars tensa is a well-ordered fibrous layer with peripheral thickening in the form of the annulus, whereas the pars flaccida is a poorly organised fibrous layer with no annulus.

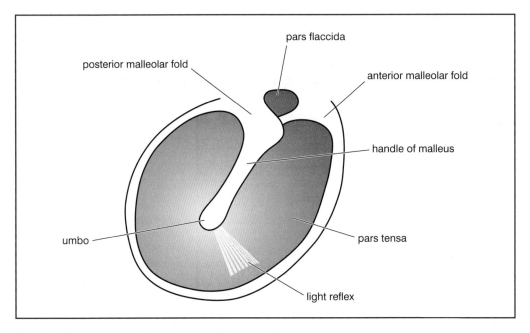

Fig. 12 The tympanic membrane (right side)

Wax in the ear is made up of secretions from sebaceous and apocrine glands and skin cells. Skin and wax normally migrates radially outwards from the tympanic membrane to the annulus and then laterally along the canal.

Otitis externa

Otitis externa is a diffuse inflammation of the skin lining the external auditory canal, and it may be bacterial or fungal. Risk factors include:

◆ getting the ears wet, perhaps through swimming
◆ trauma
◆ underlying skin disease, such as eczema
◆ diabetes.

Clinical features

◆ Moderately tender ear
◆ Discharge, which sometimes has an offensive odour
◆ Swollen canal

The discharge should be swabbed. *Staphylococcus* and *Pseudomonas* are the commonest causative organisms.

Management

◆ Topical eardrops such as gentamicin empirically.
◆ A wick or ribbon gauze may be inserted in severe infection, covered in an ointment such as Tri-Adcortyl.
◆ Therapy should be adjusted in line with swab results.
◆ Fungal infections may be treated with amphotericin or miconazole.

Malignant otitis externa

Malignant otitis externa is a severe infection, usually caused by *Pseudomonas* spp., which is characterised by bone erosion and cranial nerve paralysis. It is more common in diabetics and requires histological and CT examination to make the diagnosis. Treatment is with iv antibiotics for an extended period.

Foreign body in the ear

◆ Usually inserted by young children.
◆ May be removed by careful manipulation using a microscope if the child is co-operative; otherwise, a general anaesthetic may be indicated.
◆ The tympanic membrane should always be checked for perforation afterwards.
◆ Live insects in the ear should be killed first by oil or spirit and then removed.

Perforation

The eardrum may be perforated by direct or indirect trauma, and this will lead to:

◆ pain
◆ deafness
◆ occasionally tinnitus or vertigo.

Acute perforations should be treated with prophylactic antibiotics if direct trauma has occurred. Otherwise, no intervention is indicated other than re-inspection if hearing does not return to normal within a few weeks, as most perforations will heal themselves. If not, and a notable hearing loss is persistent, a myringoplasty may be indicated.

Tympanosclerosis

◆ Calcareous deposits on the tympanic membrane may be seen on otological examination, usually on the pars tensa.
◆ Deposits may also be present in the tympanic cavity and the mastoid.
◆ They represent an abnormal healing response to injury.
◆ They may occur after myringotomy, and the changes occur in the lamina propria of the tympanic membrane.
◆ Middle ear involvement is much less common, and it usually results in a dry perforation and significant hearing loss.

Management

◆ Conductive hearing is managed by a hearing aid.
◆ Surgery may include stapedectomy or disease clearance, although this is controversial as some think the disease recurs.

Tympanoplasty/myringoplasty

Tympanoplasty is an operation to eradicate disease from the middle ear, and to reconstruct the hearing mechanism where necessary, including reconstruction of the tympanic membrane. Myringoplasty is reconstruction of the membrane alone.

◆ Tympanoplasty techniques vary in the application of the new membrane onto the exposed middle ear bones, depending on the degree to which these bones have been eroded (Wullstein defined five techniques, and Garcia Ibanez added a sixth).
◆ The ossicles may also be reconstructed using bone autograft or porous ceramic. Malleus, incus or incudostapedius joint reconstruction may therefore be achieved.
◆ The tympanic membrane is repaired using autograft material, which may be temporal fascia, fat or cartilage; this is usually taken from behind the ear via an endoaural or postaural incision.
◆ After tympanoplasty, the patient's ear is dressed. This dressing is removed after 1–2 weeks. Exertion and flying should be avoided in the first 2 months, and scuba diving may displace any prosthesis and is contraindicated.

MIDDLE EAR

Anatomy

The middle ear (Fig. 13) contains:

◆ ossicles – malleus, incus and stapes
◆ stapedius – this acts to adjust the angle of the stapes and hence make it less sensitive to sound
◆ tensor tympani
◆ corda tympani – this part of the facial nerve communicates with the mandibular division

of the trigeminal nerve. It passes between the two layers of the tympanic membrane and over the handle of the malleus

◆ tympanic plexus of nerves – this part of the tympanic branch of the glossopharyngeal nerve joins with parasympathetic fibres of the facial nerve, and sympathetic fibres from the internal carotid artery. It ends up supplying secretomotor fibres to the parotid gland.

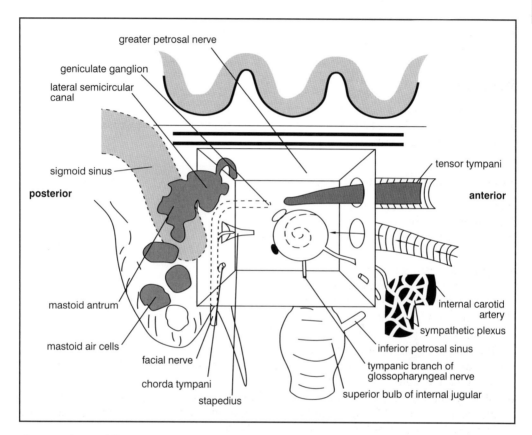

Fig. 13 The middle ear

The ossicles are arranged in such a way as to increase the force but reduce the amplitude of the sound vibrations picked up from the tympanic membrane, in a ratio of 1:21 anatomically, which translates into a physiological ratio of 1:14 in practice.

The blood supply to the middle ear is from:

◆ anterior tympanic artery from maxillary artery
◆ superior tympanic artery from middle meningeal artery
◆ posterior tympanic artery from stylomastoid artery
◆ inferior tympanic artery from ascending pharyngeal artery.

The sensory nerve supply to the middle ear is from:

- glossopharyngeal nerve via 'Jacobson's nerve'
- facial nerve.

Acute otitis media

Otitis media is an infection in the middle ear:

- common in children and frequently bilateral
- often may follow upper respiratory tract infection
- may be bacterial or viral
- *Streptococcus pneumoniae* and *Haemophilus influenzae* are the commonest causative organisms.

Clinical features

- Severe ear pain
- Hearing loss
- Temperature
- Bulging eardrum on examination
- Perforation of the drum brings relief from pain

Treatment

- Systemic or oral antibiotics, usually penicillin.
- Take a swab of any discharge.
- Surgical myringotomy may bring relief if antibiotic therapy has had no effect.

Complications

- The mastoid air cells lie close to the middle ear, and infection may spread.
- A tender swelling in the postauricular region, along with an opaque mastoid region on CT scanning are signs that iv antibiotics should be given.
- If there is no response in 24 hours, a cortical mastoidectomy may be necessary, with all air cells drilled and a drain left in situ.

Other complications of otitis media include:

- meningitis – photophobia and neck rigidity may be present
- extradural abscess – extension around the lateral sinus or above the tegmen tympani (a thin plate of bone)
- brain abscess – temporal lobe or cerebellar abscess
- subdural abscess
- lateral sinus thrombosis – ascending thrombophlebitis may cause septic emboli and metastatic abscesses; papilloedema may be present and there may be cortical signs
- facial paralysis – especially in the presence of a dehiscent facial nerve

- petrositis – spread to the petrous apex of the temporal bone may cause weakness of cranial nerves V and VI – known as Gradenigo's syndrome
- Citelli's abscess – spreads from the mastoid medially into the digastric fossa
- Bezold's abscess – spreads inferiorly in the sheath of sternocleidomastoid to form a mass on its anterior border.

Chronic otitis media

Chronic otitis media may lead to an effusion:

- Inadequate opening of the eustachian tube leads to a decrease in aeration of the middle ear.
- The remaining air is reabsorbed by the surrounding mucosa.
- There is a decrease in pressure, which acts as an irritant to the mucosa and leads to an increase in secretion.
- Eventually there is a change in the characteristics of this mucosa from flat epithelial cells to columnar ciliated mucus-producing goblet cells.
- The resultant exudates further block aeration, producing a vicious circle and leading to a hearing loss of 20–40 dB.

Long-term discharge from a perforated ear may further damage the structures of the middle ear. This may be:

- **Mucosal discharge** – signifying an underlying perforation. The discharge should be swabbed for appropriate treatment. If perforation is present it is usually in the pars tensa and central, ie there is a ring of intact tympanic membrane visible around it, and a myringoplasty may be indicated.
- **Squamous discharge** – the perforation is more likely to be postero-superior or in the pars flaccida, and involves the bony annulus. Polyps and granulations may be seen, and an underlying cholesteatoma may be present. Regular toilet is indicated in these cases, but persistence may lead to some form of atticotomy or mastoidectomy to explore and clear the underlying disease.

Ventilation tubes

Grommet insertion:

- is most commonly indicated for glue ear
- involves the insertion of a grommet in the anterior inferior portion of the tympanic membrane
- is indicated in a patient with clinical and audiometric evidence of glue ear who has not responded to a suitable period of 'wait and watch' management
- may usefully be accompanied by adenoidectomy as this may improve eustachian tube function and prevent recurrence
- is associated with tympanosclerosis in 40% 1 year after operation
- may also lead to infection, necessitating removal of the grommet

- Shah grommets self-extrude after 9 months on average – 'mini-grommets' cause less trauma but stay in for a shorter time
- T-tubes offer more permanent ventilation, but are associated with a much higher rate of residual perforation
- patients with grommets in situ should avoid getting soapy water in their ears.

Mastoidectomy

This is an operation to eradicate disease from mastoid air cells. Either an endoaural or post-aural incision is used to gain access to the attic, tegmen and sigmoid sinus. Various techniques are used:

Cortical mastoidectomy – This is used to treat acute non-cholesteatoma mastoiditis. A post-aural incision is deepened to the periosteum over the mastoid, which is then drilled to expose the mastoid air cells, leaving bone over the sigmoid sinus and middle fossa dura. Macewen's triangle is used as the landmark of the mastoid. This is made up of the temporal line superiorly, the tangent to the posterior external auditory canal posteriorly and the posterior superior rim of the canal.

Modified radical mastoidectomy – This is used for cholesteatoma. A cortical mastoid-ectomy is performed, and the wall of the posterior canal is removed to continue eradication of disease. Alternatively, the disease may be eradicated from anterior to posterior, which means that the cavity is only as big as the extent of the disease. The resultant cavity may be lined with fascia graft, or it may be obliterated using bone or muscle. Reconstruction of hearing may be considered at the same time, in the same manner as for a tympanoplasty, or may be left for a further procedure.

Combined-approach tympanoplasty – This is used for cholesteatoma. A cortical mastoid-ectomy is extended, and a posterior tympanotomy is performed so that the middle ear contents can be viewed and accessed. The canal wall is left in place and there is a risk of recurrence of cholesteatoma.

Complications

- Facial nerve damage
- Cerebrospinal fluid (CSF) leak
- Labyrinthine fistula
- Vertigo
- Damage to the ossicles

A labyrinthine fistula is **a defect in the bone that exposes the endosteum of the labyrinth**, and should not be confused with a perilymph fistula (which is defined as a perilymph leak into the middle ear arising from an oval- or round-window defect).

Symptoms

- A positive fistula sign – raising of pressure in the external ear canal causes deviation of the eyes away from the fistula.
- The Tullio phenomenon – vertigo in the presence of loud noises.

Otosclerosis

- It is an autosomal dominant disease.
- It involves the replacement of mature bone derived from the otic capsule with woven bone.
- Foci occur most commonly anterior to the oval window.
- Symptoms occur when the stapes footplate becomes fixed; 0.5–2% of the population suffer clinical symptoms as a result and 85% of these have bilateral disease.
- The male:female ratio is 2:1.

Clinical features

- Deafness
- Tinnitus
- Vertigo
- Hearing may be better in noisy surroundings – paracusis willisii
- 10% have a pink tinge on the tympanic membrane known as 'Schwartze's sign', resulting from dilated vessels on the promontory
- PTA reveals a conductive loss, with masked bone conduction demonstrating a Carhart notch, which is a dip at 2 kHz

Management

- Hearing aid.
- A stapedectomy may be indicated if the hearing loss is over 15 dB conductive.
- Women who have not completed their family should avoid the operation as the disease may progress in pregnancy.

INNER EAR

Anatomy

The inner ear (Fig. 14) consists of a labyrinth of canals embedded in the temporal bone. It can be divided into two parts:

- the vestibule and semicircular canals
- the cochlea.

The membranous labyrinth encloses a hollow system filled with endolymph, the endo-lymphatic system. The endolymph passes into a blind sac close to the sigmoid sinus, the saccus endolymphaticus. The perilymphatic system surrounds the membranous labyrinth, and communicates with the subarachnoid space via the cochlear aqueduct.

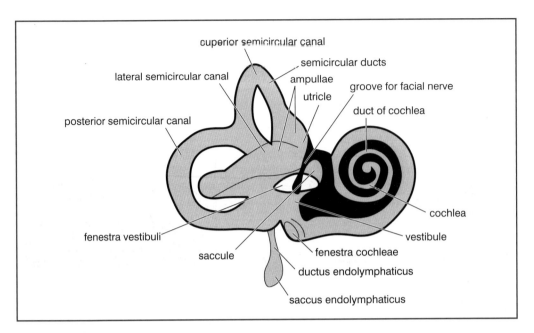

Fig. 14 The inner ear

- Perilymphatic fluid is a filtrate of blood and of CSF.
- Endolymphatic fluid in turn is a filtrate of perilymphatic fluid, but it has a different sodium and potassium concentration, due to the ion exchange system in operation.

The inner ear contains the cochlea, which is the organ of hearing:

- The cochlea consists of 2.5 turns around a bony core called the modiolus.
- There is a central cochlear duct, which contains endolymph.
- The endolymph transmits vibrations to the tectorial membrane.
- This leads to movement of the underlying hair cells, which causes changes in polarisation via alterations in potassium permeability.
- There is a consequent transmission of information to the cochlear nerve.

The cochlear duct is sandwiched between the scala vestibuli and the scala tympani, both of which contain perilymph (Fig. 15). The upper and lower separating boundaries are known as the 'vestibular membrane' and the 'basilar membrane', respectively. The vestibular membrane is also known as 'Reissner's membrane'.

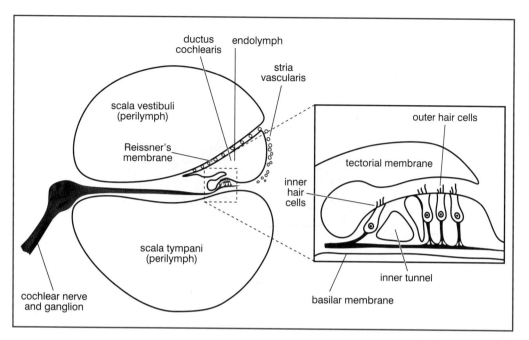

Fig. 15 Cross-section of the cochlea

The inner ear also contains three semicircular canals:

♦ The canals are arranged at right angles to each other.
♦ Each includes a widening known as an 'ampulla'.
♦ Each ampulla contains a gelatinous mass known as the 'cupula', which surrounds a collection of hair cells embedded in the underlying membrane (Fig. 16).
♦ Movement of the surrounding endolymph caused by rotatory motion leads to movement of the cupula and of the hair cells.
♦ The cells are depolarised and transmit impulses to the vestibular nerves.
♦ The saccule acts in a similar way to detect linear accelerations and decelerations, and the utricle acts to detect gravity.
♦ These vestibular organs are responsible for about 15% of balance function, and their outputs are integrated with proprioceptive (15%) and visual (70%) outputs to be integrated in the brainstem to maintain balance.

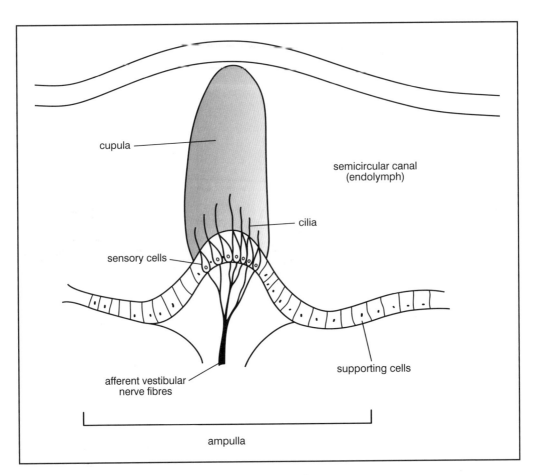

Fig. 16 Ampulla and cupula of a semicircular canal

These structures are all contained within the temporal bone, which consists of a number of parts (Fig. 17):

◆ squamous temporal bone
◆ petrous temporal bone
◆ stylomastoid foramen
◆ inner auditory meatus
◆ mastoid bone
◆ styloid process.

SECTION 1

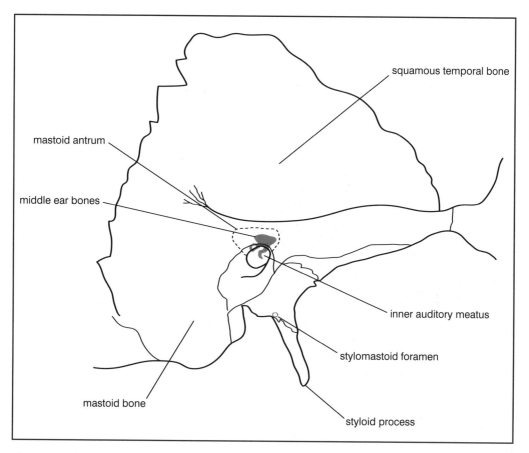

Fig. 17 Right temporal bone

The inner auditory meatus exits on the posterior fossa surface of the temporal bone. The anterior half contains the facial nerve above and the cochlear nerve below, and the posterior half contains the superior and inferior vestibular nerves.

Temporal bone fractures

- **Longitudinal** – 80% of fractures have a dominant longitudinal component, usually from a lateral skull blow. The tympanic membrane may be torn and there may be a haemo-tympanum or CSF leak. Facial nerve injury is not common.
- **Transverse** – these dominate in 20%, from an anterior or posterior blow. The tympanic membrane is usually intact, and there may be facial nerve damage, sensorineural hearing loss, vertigo and cranial nerve injury.

A history of immediate facial nerve palsy after head injury may indicate the need for surgical decompression of the nerve. A delayed palsy may resolve with conservative management.

Auditory pathway

Once generated, the auditory information is transmitted via the auditory pathway to the cerebral cortex. This can be summarised as follows:

◆ cochlear nerve
◆ synapses in cochlear nuclei in the medulla
◆ crosses to contralateral side

◆ passes through nucleus of the trapezoid body and superior olivary nucleus in the brainstem
◆ passes upwards through the nucleus of lateral lemniscus
◆ reaches the inferior colliculus
◆ passes to the medial geniculate body of the thalamus and synapses
◆ final neurone passes to the cerebral cortex.

Stapedectomy

◆ Otosclerosis is the commonest indication.
◆ It involves the creation of a fenestra to remove the fixed portion of the stapes footplate.
◆ This fenestra may be:
  ● small – formed with the aid of micro-instruments or a laser
  ● large – involving removal of a large part of the stapes footplate.
◆ The oval window is then usually sealed with vein graft.
◆ A prosthesis is inserted to close the air–bone gap.
◆ The patient should be warned about the risks of a dead ear, vertigo and alteration to the sense of taste, as well as damage to the facial nerve.
◆ Complications include tympanosclerosis, a floating or depressed footplate, saccular injury, perilymph fistula, displacement of the prosthesis and necrosis of the incus.

Ménière's disease

The aetiology of this condition is still unknown, although it is thought that an expansion of the endolymphatic fluid volume results in pressure on the basilar membrane and eventually leads to rupture of Reissner's membrane.

Clinical features

◆ Episodic tinnitus
◆ Episodic nausea and vertigo
◆ Deafness, classically high-frequency
◆ Attacks last a few hours
◆ Often there is a prodromal warning phase

Patients are at first normal in between attacks, and their vertiginous symptoms improve with time, although hearing will eventually show a permanent deterioration. This is classically a low-frequency hearing loss. Electrocochleography and caloric tests may provide further evidence. The triad of episodic vertigo, tinnitus and deafness is sometimes described as **Ménière's syndrome**, and may have another cause, such as acoustic neuroma.

Management

◆ Treatment is controversial.
◆ Medical treatment may include reduced salt and fluid intake.
◆ Betahistine and vestibular sedatives may help.
◆ Medical treatment may result in improvement in 80% of patients.
◆ Surgical treatment:
  ● decompression of the endolymphatic sac
  ● vestibular nerve section
  ● vestibular labyrinth destruction via gentamicin
  ● surgical labyrinthectomy may be indicated in very severe cases.

Vertigo

Vertigo is defined as the **hallucination of movement**. A detailed history must be taken from any patient presenting with vertigo to determine the exact nature of the problem and any precipitating or relieving factors. Vestibular causes of vertigo can be divided in two groups:

◆ **Central causes** – cerebrovascular accident/migraine/tumours/multiple sclerosis may all compromise the vestibular nuclei in the brainstem, due to vascular insufficiency, nerve demyelination or pressure effects on the brain. Cervical vertigo may occur, and this is thought to be due to a confused interpretation of proprioceptive information from the neck. Drugs may also have a central effect.
◆ **Peripheral causes** – the peripheral vestibular system may be affected by three main pathologies:
  ● **Benign positional vertigo** may occur after a head injury or ear infection and is brought on by a particular head movement. Hallpike's manoeuvre is diagnostic, and Epley's manoeuvre or Brandt–Daroff exercises may work as a treatment.
  ● **Ménière's disease** is thought to be due to excess pressure of endolymphatic fluid in the vestibular canals and is accompanied by tinnitus and temporary hearing loss, lasting from minutes to hours. Dietary restrictions may help, and treatment with betahistine is successful in some patients; acute episodes may be treated by antiemetics.
  ● **Acute vestibular failure** may be brought on by an upper respiratory tract infection and may last for many days. Treatment is largely symptomatic.

Other causes of peripheral vestibular dysfunction include cholesteatoma and acoustic neuroma.

4 Rhinology

ANATOMY AND PHYSIOLOGY OF THE NOSE

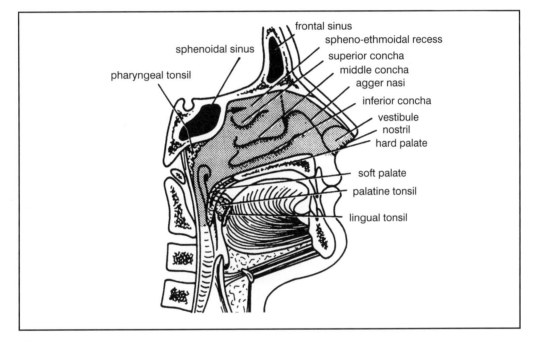

Fig. 18 Anatomy of the nose

The nose consists of:

◆ the external nose, made up of cartilage
◆ two nasal cavities made up of nasal bones and separated by the bony and cartilaginous septum
◆ two posterior choanae, leading to the nasopharynx.

Air flows in and out of the lungs through the nose and nasopharynx. The nose:

◆ warms
◆ moistens, and
◆ filters incoming air.

The nasal mucosa undergoes a **reflex nasal cycle**, in which, every 2–6 hours, one lumen of the nose widens due to vasodilatation in mucosa, while the other narrows, giving a constant airway resistance. Also, pressure in the crook of the arm (Eccles' reflex) or lying on one side of the body causes the contralateral airway to open. The purpose of these reflexes is not fully understood.

Most of the nasal cavity is lined with columnar ciliated respiratory epithelium, apart from the area of the olfactory cleft and cribriform plate known as the **olfactory region**:

◆ The olfactory region is lined with olfactory mucosa.
◆ It is innervated by bipolar fibres of the olfactory nerve.
◆ About 20 fibres run to the primary olfactory centre of the olfactory bulb.
◆ Fibres travel via the olfactory tract to the secondary olfactory centre.
◆ Eventually they reach the dentate and semilunate gyri in the cerebral cortex.
◆ Olfactory nerve fibres are surrounded by supporting cells.
◆ A lipid secretion in this area aids differentiation of odours.

EXTERNAL NOSE AND VESTIBULE

Anatomy

The external nose and nasal vestibule are largely made up of cartilage (Fig. 19):

◆ bilateral greater alar cartilages laterally, containing a lateral and a medial crus
◆ lateral nasal cartilage on both sides
◆ cartilaginous nasal septum.

The resultant horse-shoe shape at the entrance to the nose forms the nasal vestibule on either side. In the midline the connective tissue columella lies below the septum. The sensory nerve supply is from the first two branches of the trigeminal nerve.

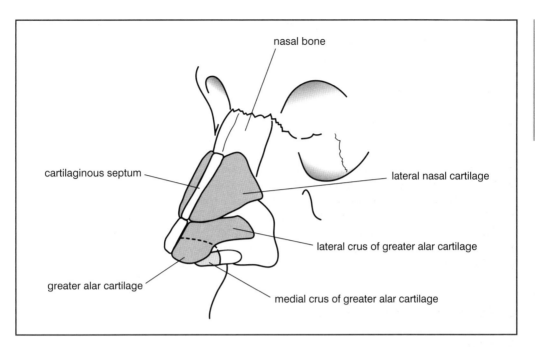

Fig. 19 The nasal cartilages

The junction between the nasal vestibule and the nasal cavity is known as the **internal nasal valve**:

- It is the narrowest part of the nasal airway.
- It may be the rate-limiting point for airflow.
- It is largely made up of the anterior edge of the lateral nasal cartilage.

Trauma

Nasal trauma is commonly due to assault, road traffic accidents, sports or falls. Fracture of the nasal bone may be accompanied by complications:

- Septal haematomas usually present as a cherry-red swelling in the mucoperichondrium of the septum. If bilateral, incision and drainage is required to prevent re-accumulation and consequent destruction of the cartilage.
- Presence of watery rhinorrhoea indicates possible fracture of the cribriform plate and the need for antibiotic coverage to prevent meningitis. Some leaks require formal surgical closure with temporalis fascia.

Management

- Check airway patency, presence of epistaxis, septal haematoma, ocular movements and trigeminal nerve sensation, and stabilise the patient as appropriate.

- Simple nasal fractures require a second assessment 5–7 days after the oedema has regressed.
- Manipulation under anaesthesia may be necessary and this should be done no more than 2 weeks after the initial injury, or the bones may set in position.
- If septal damage is present, removal of the damaged part is necessary and, if the septum has collapsed, an open reduction may be necessary.
- If these methods fail and the bone subsequently sets, a septorhinoplasty will be required for correction.

Nasal fracture manipulation

Manipulation is indicated if a fracture of the nasal bones is clinically evident. Reduction may be achieved under a general anaesthetic by simple lateral pressure or with the use of instruments such as Walshingham's forceps to realign the bone fragments. A plaster cast over the nose may be necessary to keep the adjusted bones in place during healing.

Complications

- No improvement
- Bleeding
- Pain
- Setting of the fracture in an unsatisfactory position, requiring septorhinoplasty

NASAL CAVITY

Anatomy

The nasal cavity proper is largely made up of bone. Various cranial bones are involved, and these can be seen in a medial section through the nose in Fig. 20.

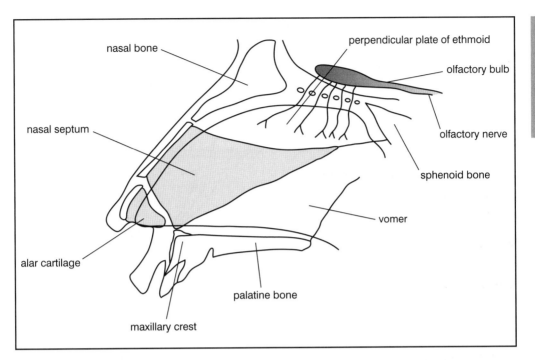

Fig. 20 The medial nasal wall

The lateral wall of the nasal cavity (Fig. 21) has three turbinates on either side – bony ridges that are thought to increase the surface area of the nasal mucosa. Ostia of all the sinuses apart from the sphenoid sinus are located on the lateral wall, as well as the opening of the nasolacrimal duct. The superior, middle and inferior meatuses lie inferior to the three turbinates.

- ◆ Superior meatus – this contains the opening of the posterior ethmoid sinus and, behind this, the opening of the sphenoid sinus.
- ◆ Middle meatus – this contains the openings of the nasofrontal duct, anterior ethmoid sinus and maxillary antrum.
- ◆ Inferior meatus – this contains the opening of the nasolacrimal duct.

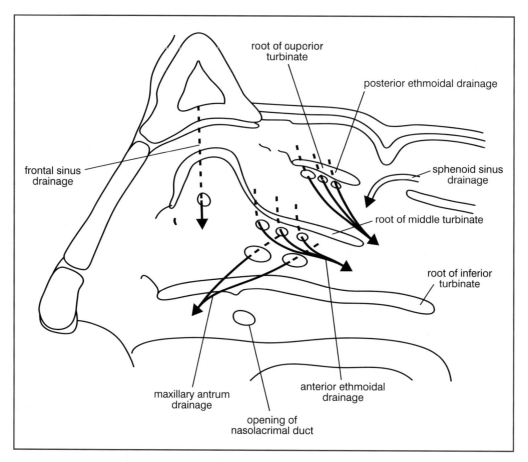

Fig. 21 The lateral nasal wall

Blood supply of the medial nasal wall (Fig. 22):

◆ Little's area, also known as 'Kiesselbach's area', is particularly rich in small vessels supplied by both internal and external carotid arteries.

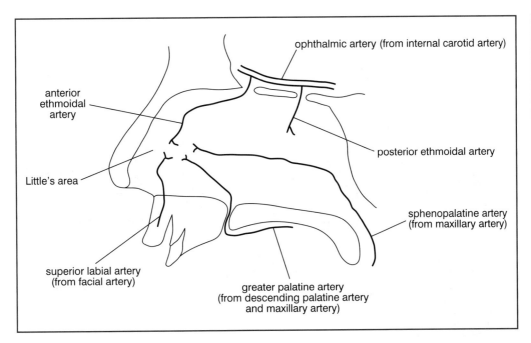

Fig. 22 Blood supply of medial nasal wall

Nerve supply of the nasal cavity:

◆ Sensory nerve supply for the nasal cavity and sinuses is provided by the first and second branches of the trigeminal nerves, as well as the olfactory nerve.
◆ Sympathetic and parasympathetic nerve supply is complex:
  ● Sympathetic supply travels from the T1–T5 segments to the superior cervical ganglion, where it synapses. It then travels via the blood vessels to the nasal mucosa.
  ● Parasympathetic supply travels from the superior salivary nucleus to the geniculate ganglion, and thence along the facial nerve, the greater superficial petrosal nerve and the nerve of the pterygoid canal (vidian nerve) to the pterygopalatine ganglion. Here it synapses and runs to the mucosa.

Foreign body

◆ Usually self-inserted by 2–3-year-old children.
◆ May remain in place for a long time.
◆ May only be noticed when a foul smell and chronic rhinitis begins.
◆ Unilateral rhinitis should arouse suspicion of a foreign body.
◆ Removal is sometimes possible by blowing in the contralateral nostril with patient's mouth closed.
◆ The next stage is removal via instrumentation, if necessary under an anaesthetic.
◆ Bleeding and infection may be present.
◆ Nasal foreign bodies should be removed relatively urgently because of the danger of aspiration.

Epistaxis

Epistaxis is usually harmless, but may be life threatening. Most bleeding originates in Little's area (see above). A concise history, taking note of risk factors such as use of warfarin and hypertension, should be taken.

Causes of epistaxis

Local

◆ Idiopathic
◆ Traumatic
◆ Iatrogenic
◆ Foreign body
◆ Bleeding polyp
◆ Tumours of the nose or nasopharynx, eg nasopharyngeal angiofibroma

Systemic

◆ Vascular diseases such as hypertension
◆ Coagulopathies such as haemophilia
◆ Thrombopathies such as idiopathic thrombocytopenic purpura, sickle cell anaemia
◆ Vasculopathies such as Henoch–Schönlein purpura (HSP)
◆ Hereditary haemorrhagic telangiectasia (HHT, Osler–Weber–Rendu disease) leads to multifocal bleeding from the septum

---

Management

◆ History taking is followed by localisation of the bleeding, which can generally be categorised as anterior or posterior.
◆ Conservative measures may be tried, such as ice packs and nasal alae pressure.
◆ Continuing anterior bleeding may then be treated directly with a local anaesthetic spray and cautery with silver nitrate sticks or diathermy.
◆ It is important to bear in mind that only one side of the nasal septum should be cauterised at a time, as bilateral cautery leaves the septal cartilage with no blood supply.
◆ The patient should be sitting up, and they should be nursed in a calm but well-lit environment. The doctor should have all necessary equipment to hand.
◆ In cases of severe bleeding, priority should be given to inserting an iv line; make preparations for blood transfusion if necessary.
◆ If cautery is impossible or unsuccessful, anterior bleeding may be arrested by the use of a nasal tampon or packing.
◆ Posterior bleeding may require a posterior pack or balloon catheter.
◆ The contralateral nostril may need to be packed.
◆ Posterior balloon catheters should not apply pressure on the nasal alae or columella as necrosis may quickly result.

Aftercare

◆ After stabilisation, any contributing factors such as warfarin overdose or hypertension should be treated.
◆ Moisturisation of the nasal mucosa with aqueous gel may be helpful in preventing recurrences.
◆ Use of a postnasal balloon or pack requires coverage with antibiotics due to the consequent obstruction of the eustachian tube.

For intractable or recurrent bleeding, operative measures may be necessary. Vascular ligation under a general anaesthetic is possible, and the following arteries may be ligated:

◆ sphenopalatine artery – this is accessed endoscopically at the rear of the middle turbinate
◆ internal maxillary artery – this is accessed in the pterygopalatine fossa via a Caldwell–Luc incision and posterior window in the antrum
◆ anterior and posterior ethmoidal arteries – these are accessed externally via a medial orbital incision
◆ external carotid artery – this is accessed at the anterior border of sternocleidomastoid.

A septoplasty may be necessary if a troublesome bone spur is impeding access to the bleeding point. Patients with HHT may require treatment by split-skin grafts, laser therapy or radiotherapy to reduce the incidence of bleeding.

Rhinitis

Rhinitis is inflammation of the nasal mucosa and can be divided simply into allergic and intrinsic rhinitis.

Allergic rhinitis – This is a type I hypersensitivity reaction, and it can be seasonal or perennial. It occurs in response to proteins or glycoproteins such as pollens, moulds and house dust mites. Rhinorrhoea, sneezing and nasal irritation are present and the nasal mucosa is moist, pale and swollen. Skin-prick tests may reveal allergens, as may plasma IgE testing, although avoidance of the allergen is not always possible. Oral antihistamine and topical steroid sprays are mostly used in treatment, as well as topical anticholinergics and sodium cromoglycate.

Intrinsic rhinitis – This is generally thought to be a diagnosis of exclusion, with no identifiable trigger. Nasal polyps are common, with nasal obstruction and discharge. Many patients have sinus pathology. The nasal mucosa is red and irritated. Medical treatment is similar to that of allergic rhinitis but surgical treatment is more helpful – polypectomy, turbinate reduction, vidian neurectomy (hence cutting off the parasympathetic supply, although the condition seems to relapse quickly) and functional endoscopic sinus surgery (FESS).

Septoplasty

1 Septoplasty may be indicated to improve nasal airway and breathing.
2 Local anaesthetic is injected deep to the nasal septal mucosa, which aids dissection.
3 An incision is made at the front of the nasal septum (hemi-transfixion or Killian's).
4 The nasal mucosa is lifted from the underlying cartilage to reach the perpendicular plate of the ethmoid and the vomer.
5 Adjustments are made to the septal cartilage, the perpendicular bone and the maxillary crest so that the septum lies straight.
6 Care is taken not to remove structures too anteriorly as this causes saddle-nose deformity.
7 Turbinate reduction surgery may also be performed.

Complications

◆ Bleeding
◆ Saddle-nose deformity
◆ No resolution of presenting complaint
◆ Septal perforation

Rhinoplasty

Rhinoplasty may be combined with septoplasty and is indicated for cosmetic reasons and to improve the airway. It is important to clarify what the patient dislikes about their nose before operating and not to give the patient unrealistic expectations of the result. The operation may utilise various techniques, in particular nasal dehumping, osteotomies and lower lateral cartilage rotation. Grafting may be necessary to change the cartilage profile.

Complications

◆ Bleeding
◆ Perforation
◆ Worsening of appearance
◆ Periorbital haematoma

Wegener's granulomatosis

◆ This is a disease causing destructive lesions in the upper and lower respiratory tracts and glomerulonephritis, with granuloma formation and necrotising vasculitis.
◆ It is thought to be triggered by an immunological reaction to infection.
◆ Commonly presents to ENT with nasal symptoms.
◆ In the nose there is sanguinous discharge, crust formation and ulcerated mucosa.
◆ It may also cause external and middle ear damage.
◆ Diagnosis can only made by biopsy.
◆ Cytoplasmic antineutrophilic cytoplasmic antibodies (cANCA) tend to be positive in Wegener's granulomatosis.

◆ Low-dose antibiotics are indicated, as well as the use of immunosuppressive treatment, such as with steroids or cyclophosphamide.

NASAL SINUSES

Anatomy

The functions of the sinuses are unclear but possibilities are:

◆ to decrease the weight of the skull
◆ to provide a distinctive facial shape
◆ to act as resonators for the voice.

Each sinus ostium is lined with erectile tissue, which may influence its patency.

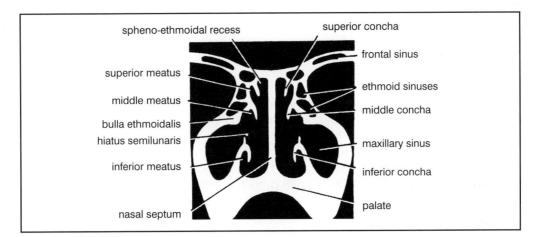

Fig. 23 The paranasal sinuses

Maxillary sinus

◆ This is the largest, with usually only one cavity on each side.
◆ Superior wall is the floor of the orbit.
◆ Posterior wall lies in front of the pterygopalatine fossa.
◆ The floor is related to the roots of the maxillary teeth.
◆ Maxillary sinuses are usually small until after the seventh year.
◆ Nerve supply – anterior, middle and posterior superior alveolar nerves (ie from the maxillary nerve).

Frontal sinus

◆ This is divided into right and left, often different in size.
◆ Floor forms part of the roof of the orbit.

- Posterior wall forms part of the bony anterior cranial fossa, giving potential for intracranial complications.
- Nerve supply – supraorbital nerve (from the ophthalmic nerve).

Ethmoid sinuses

- Six to ten air-containing cells; may be divided into anterior and posterior cells.
- The superior wall forms the anterior skull base.
- The lateral wall forms the lamina papyracea, which separates the sinus from the orbital cavity.
- Nerve supply – anterior and posterior branches of the nasociliary nerve.

Sphenoid sinus

- This lies in the skull base in the body of the sphenoid bone.
- The superior wall is related to the anterior and middle cranial fossae, as well as the optic chiasma, optic foramen, and sella turcica with the pituitary gland.
- The lateral walls are related to the cavernous sinuses, cranial nerves II–IV and the internal carotid artery.
- The posterior wall is very thick, and behind it lies the posterior cranial fossa and the pons.
- Nerve supply – posterior ethmoidal nerve.

Sinusitis

Any blockage of the drainage passages may lead to stasis of secretions in the sinuses, and consequent infection. This may be caused by polyps, anatomical variation, rhinitis, and upper respiratory tract infections, as well as mucociliary disorders such as Kartagener's syndrome or cystic fibrosis.

Acute sinusitis

- This mostly affects the maxillary sinuses.
- Stasis and secondary bacterial infection most commonly is with *Streptococcus pneumoniae* or *Haemophilus influenzae*.
- Acute fungal sinusitis may also be present.
- Facial pain and pyrexia may result, and there may be pus visible in the middle meatus on nasoendoscopy.
- Treatment is with broad-spectrum antibiotics and a decongestant such as pseudoephedrine.
- Local treatment of the middle meatus with a cocaine-soaked pledget may also be carried out.
- If there is no response to this medical treatment, FESS surgery, antrostomy, frontal sinus trephine, anterior sphenoidotomy or ethmoidectomy may be necessary.

Chronic sinusitis

◆ Symptoms persist for weeks to months.
◆ Granulation tissue, ulceration of the epithelium and mucosal thickening may all become irreversible with time.
◆ Medical treatment with antibiotics and decongestants should also be tried in these patients.
◆ FESS and open sinus surgery are employed in intractable cases.

Fungal sinusitis

This may be divided into the following categories:

◆ Allergic fungal sinusitis – associated with nasal polyps and asthma; steroids and itraconazole may be used.
◆ Mycetoma – masses of fungal debris are present in the sinuses; surgical removal is indicated.
◆ Acute invasive – occurs in immunocompromised patients and requires radical debridement.
◆ Chronic indolent – most commonly due to *Aspergillus*; surgical debridement is required.

Nasal polyps

Nasal polyps are **herniations of nasal mucosa**, caused by oedema of the connective tissue, which contains an eosinophilic infiltrate. Symptoms include:

◆ obstruction
◆ discharge
◆ anosmia
◆ widening of the distance between the medial corners of the eyes.

Management

◆ Intranasal steroids.
◆ Antihistamines may be helpful.
◆ Surgery may be used to remove the polyps, although they have a high rate of recurrence.
◆ Suspicious-looking polyps, or unilateral lesions, should be sent for histological examination to exclude neoplasia.
◆ Antro-choanal polyps are large, often unilateral polyps, originating in the maxillary antrum and prolapsing through into the nasal cavity; endoscopic treatment is usually successful, but an open Caldwell–Luc procedure may be necessary.

Sinonasal tumours

Sinonasal tumours may present late, as they may grow substantially before symptoms present.

Benign tumours

◆ **Inverted papilloma** – presents as a papillomatous mass in the nose, with microscopic invaginations of epithelium into stroma. Surgical excision and careful follow-up is required, as there may be a nasal carcinoma as well. A lateral rhinotomy is often necessary for excision.
◆ **Osteoma** – commonest in the frontal regions and made up of cortical bone.

Malignant tumours

◆ 50% are squamous cell carcinomas – cigarette smoking is the biggest risk factor.
◆ 15% are anaplastic.
◆ 10% are lymphomas.
◆ 4% are adenocarcinomas – hardwood workers are at risk.

Other malignant tumours

◆ **Olfactory neuroblastoma** – involving the cribriform plate and removed via a craniofacial resection.
◆ **Malignant melanoma** – usually from septum or lateral nasal wall.

Functional endoscopic sinus surgery (FESS)

This is minimally invasive surgery, and it is indicated for:

◆ rhinosinusitis
◆ polyps
◆ arrest of epistaxis
◆ repair of CSF leaks
◆ orbital decompression
◆ dacryocystorhinostomy
◆ optic nerve decompression
◆ pituitary surgery.

CT scanning is required to identify the anatomy. Surgery may be performed with cutting instruments or a microdebrider. Care must be taken not to cause too much scarring or bone damage in the operation, as this will lead to problems with healing and also difficulty in performing revisions.

Complications

- ◆ CSF leak (should be repaired immediately if possible with turbinate tissue)
- ◆ Intraorbital bleeding (may require orbital decompression)
- ◆ Nasolacrimal duct injury
- ◆ Carotid artery injury
- ◆ Optic nerve injury

5 Head and Neck/Laryngology/ Pharyngology

EMBRYOLOGY OF THE HEAD AND NECK

The **pharyngeal arches** (Table 6) consist of mesoderm, endoderm and ectoderm, and each has its own arterial and nerve supply.

Pharyngeal arch	Nerve supply	Derivatives	Muscles
First	Mandibular branch of cranial nerve V	Incus, malleus, maxilla, zygoma, part of temporal bone, mandible	Temporalis, masseter, pterygoids, anterior belly of digastric, tensor palati, tensor tympani, mylohyoid
Second	Facial nerve	Stapes, styloid process, lesser horn and upper half of hyoid, stylohyoid ligament	Muscles of facial expression, posterior belly of digastric, stapedius, stylohyoid
Third	Glossopharyngeal nerve	Greater horn and lower half of hyoid, stylopharyngeus	
Fourth and sixth	Fourth – superior laryngeal nerve Sixth – right laryngeal nerve	Laryngeal cartilage, cricothyroid, pharyngeal constrictors, levator veli palatini, intrinsic muscles of larynx	

Table 6 Overview of the pharyngeal arches

The **pharyngeal pouches** are out-pouches along the lateral pharyngeal wall; there are five pairs. The endoderm lining these pouches gives rise to various structures (Table 7).

Pharyngeal pouch	Derivatives from endoderm
First	Middle ear cavity, eustachian tube
Second	Palatine tonsils
Third	Inferior parathyroid gland, thymus
Fourth	Superior parathyroid gland
Fifth	Parafollicular (C) cells

Table 7 Derivatives of the endoderm of the pharyngeal pouches

THE NECK

Anatomy

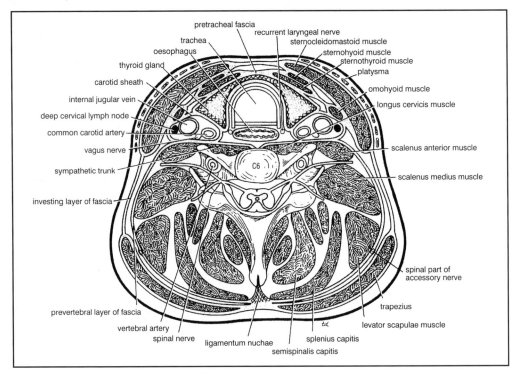

Fig. 24 Fascial layers of the neck

The neck contains various layers of fascia (Fig. 24) that divide it into different compartments:

◆ Investing fascia – extends from the base of the skull and lower border of the mandible to the spine of the scapula, lateral part of the clavicle and sternum. It splits into two layers to form the parotid fascia and also forms the stylomandibular ligament.

◆ Prevertebral fascia – lies in front of the prevertebral muscles and covers the muscles forming the floor of the posterior triangle. The accessory nerve lies superficial to this fascia.

◆ Pretracheal fascia – splits to enclose the thyroid gland and provides a slippery surface for the trachea to move during swallowing. It blends with the carotid sheath laterally.

◆ Carotid sheath – surrounds the internal jugular vein, common carotid artery and the vagus nerve. It consists of loose areolar tissue, which allows expansion of the internal jugular vein.

Anterior triangle of the neck

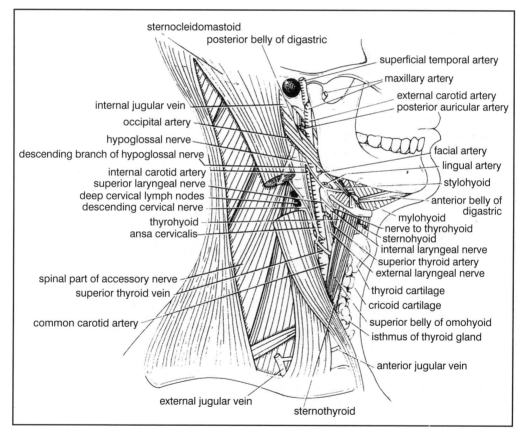

Fig. 25 Anterior triangle of the neck

Boundaries

◆ Medial – the midline
◆ Lateral – anterior border of sternocleidomastoid
◆ Superior – lower border of the mandible
◆ Roof – investing fascia
◆ Floor – prevertebral fascia

Muscles

◆ Suprahyoid muscles – digastric (V, VII), stylohyoid (VII), geniohyoid (C1), mylohyoid (V)
◆ Infrahyoid (strap) muscles – thyrohyoid (C1), sternohyoid, omohyoid, sternothyroid (all three ansa cervicalis C1/2/3 via XII)

The anterior neck is divided into the following regions:

◆ Submental triangle – submental lymph nodes, anterior jugular vein.
◆ Carotid triangle (all contents in carotid sheath) – common carotid artery, internal carotid artery, external carotid artery and branches, internal jugular vein and tributaries, hypoglossal nerve and descending branch, internal and external laryngeal nerves, deep cervical lymph nodes, accessory nerve, vagus nerve.
◆ Digastric (submandibular) triangle – submandibular salivary gland, facial artery, facial vein, submandibular lymph nodes, hypoglossal nerve, hypoglossus muscle, nerve and vessels to mylohyoid, carotid sheath, stylopharyngeus, glossopharyngeal nerve, parotid gland.
◆ Muscular triangle – sternohyoid muscle, sternothyroid muscle, thyroid gland, larynx, trachea, oesophagus.

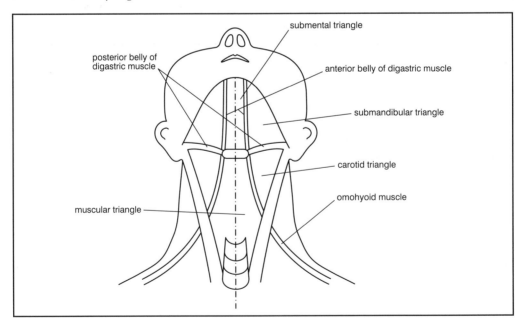

Fig. 26 Anterior neck regions

Posterior triangle of the neck

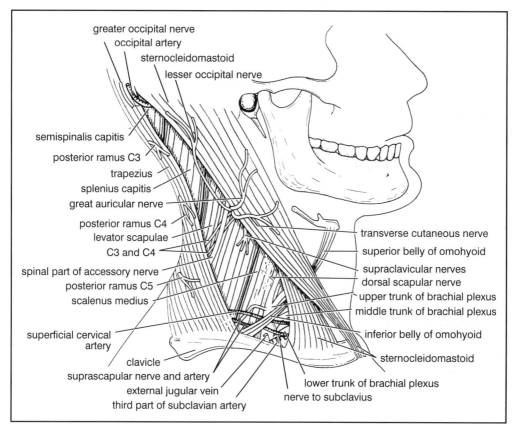

Fig. 27 Posterior triangle of the neck

Boundaries

◆ Anterior – posterior edge of sternocleidomastoid
◆ Posterior – anterior edge of trapezius
◆ Base – middle third of clavicle
◆ Roof – investing fascia
◆ Floor – prevertebral fascia overlying prevertebral muscles (splenius capitus, levator scapulae, scalenus anterior, middle and posterior).

Contents

◆ Accessory nerve
◆ Lymph nodes
◆ Occipital artery
◆ Inferior belly of omohyoid

- External jugular vein
- Transverse cervical and suprascapular vessels
- Cutaneous branches of the cervical plexus; lesser occipital, greater auricular, transverse cervical, suprascapular nerves

The surface marking of the accessory nerve is the line joining the midpoint of the posterior border of sternocleidomastoid to the anterior border of trapezius, 5 cm above the clavicle. The subclavian artery and trunks of the brachial plexus lie deep to the prevertebral fascia.

Neck space infections

Retropharyngeal abscess

From the base of the skull to the diaphragm, anterior to the prevertebral fascia, is a potential space. An abscess in this area can track to fill any part of this space, but the region behind the pharynx is most frequently affected, leading to a retropharyngeal abscess. Clinical features include:

- occurs mostly in young children, often after an upper respiratory tract infection
- neck held rigid
- systemically unwell
- airway/swallowing difficulties
- widened retropharynx on lateral X-ray
- treatment with iv antibiotics – intraluminal incision and drainage may be necessary.

Parapharyngeal abscess

The potential space lateral to the oro- and nasopharynx is divided into anterior and posterior compartments by the styloid process. The posterior compartment contains the carotid sheath. An abscess may be present in this area. Clinically:

- features are similar to peritonsillar abscess – trismus, palate oedema, throat swelling
- swelling is behind the upper posterior sternocleidomastoid
- severe complications may occur, eg internal carotid artery rupture and jugular vein thrombosis
- treatment is with iv antibiotics and repeated needle aspiration.

Submandibular abscess

The space between the mylohyoid muscle and floor of the mouth may become infected, usually secondary to dental infection; this is also known as 'Ludwig's angina'. Clinical features include:

- history of dental pain
- floor of mouth oedema and pain

- tongue pushed posteriorly
- airway compromise
- dribbling
- treatment with iv antibiotics and needle aspiration with airway protection via naso-pharyngeal tube.

Neck lumps

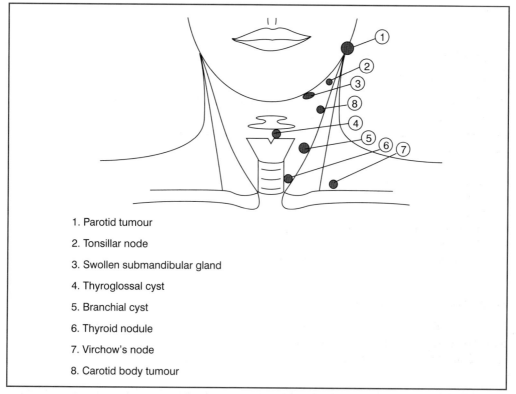

1. Parotid tumour

2. Tonsillar node

3. Swollen submandibular gland

4. Thyroglossal cyst

5. Branchial cyst

6. Thyroid nodule

7. Virchow's node

8. Carotid body tumour

Fig. 28 Lumps in the neck

Treatment

- Parotid tumour – discussed below.
- Tonsillar node – treat the tonsillitis.
- Swollen submandibular gland – discussed below.
- Thyroglossal cyst – this lies along the track of the obliterated thyroglossal tract, and may contain elements of thyroid tissue. It moves with both swallowing and tongue protrusion. Sistrunk's operation involves excision of the whole of the tract, together with the median third of the hyoid bone; there is a 10% recurrence rate.
- Branchial cyst – this is a remnant of the cervical sinus, formed from the second, third and fourth branchial grooves embryologically. It commonly presents in the third

decade. A fistula to the skin may be present. Excision of the cyst and fistula may be indicated, especially if there is infection.

Neck lymph nodes

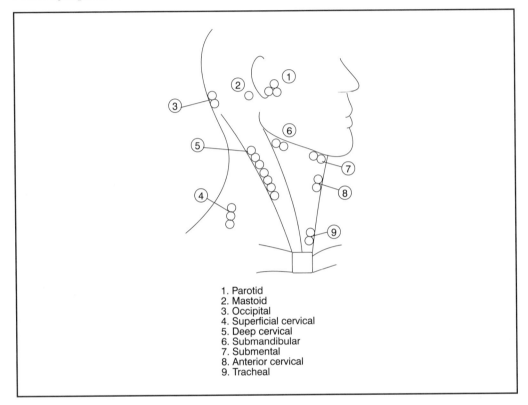

1. Parotid
2. Mastoid
3. Occipital
4. Superficial cervical
5. Deep cervical
6. Submandibular
7. Submental
8. Anterior cervical
9. Tracheal

Fig. 29 Neck lymph nodes

Node	Drains
Parotid	Scalp, face, parotid gland
Mastoid	Scalp, auricle
Occipital	Scalp
Superficial cervical (along external jugular vein)	Breast, lung, viscera, face, parotid
Deep cervical (along internal jugular vein)	All neck nodes ultimately drain to here
Submandibular	Tongue
Submental	Atrium and floor of the mouth, lips
Anterior cervical	Oesophagus, front of neck
Tracheal	Thyroid

Table 8 Lymph nodes of the neck

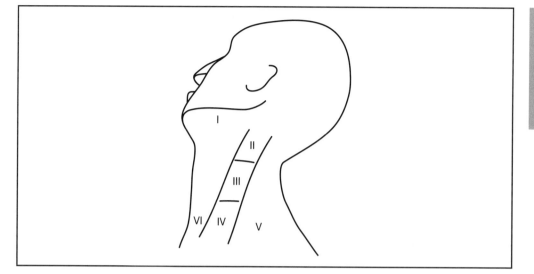

Fig. 30 Cervical lymph node levels (see text for details)

Cervical node levels (Fig. 30)

I – Submental and submandibular area between the digastric muscles and mandible
II – Around upper third of the internal jugular vein (from skull base to carotid bifurcation)
III – Around middle third of the internal jugular vein (from carotid bifurcation to cricothyroid notch)
IV – Around lower third of the internal jugular vein (form cricothyroid notch to clavicle)
V – Posterior triangle nodes
VI – Anterior compartment around trachea

Neck dissection

Removal of neck nodes may be necessary in head and neck carcinoma to reduce the chance of recurrence. The types of neck dissection are:

♦ Radical neck dissection – includes removal of submental, submandibular, jugular and posterior triangle neck nodes, as well as submandibular gland, spinal accessory nerve, internal jugular vein, and sternocleidomastoid muscle. Complications include bleeding, leak of chyle, cranial nerve palsies, and facial and cerebral oedema.
♦ Modified radical neck dissection – this is indicated if the nodes are no more than 3 cm in size. It involves removal of levels I–V cervical nodes, with preservation of at least one of internal jugular vein, accessory nerve or sternocleidomastoid. May reduce cerebral oedema in bilateral neck dissections.

♦ Selective neck dissection – this is the removal of selected levels of cervical nodes, depending on the site of origin of the tumour.
♦ Extended radical neck dissection.

PHARYNX AND ORAL CAVITY

Anatomy

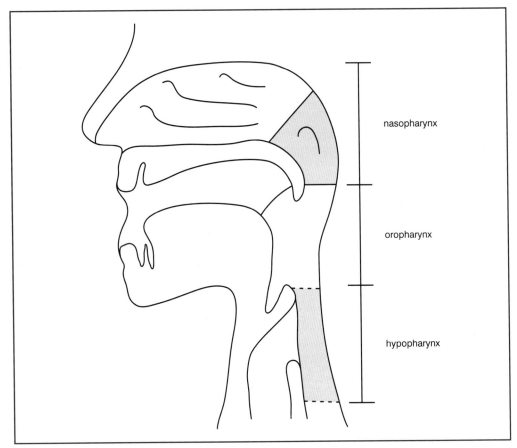

Fig. 31 Boundaries of the pharynx

Boundaries

♦ Oral cavity – this extends from the lips to the anterior faucial arch, bounded below by the floor of the mouth and above by the hard and soft palate.
♦ Nasopharynx – the superior boundary is the base of the skull; inferior boundary is an imaginary line level with the soft palate; anterior border is formed by the choanae, posterior border by the adenoid tissue; and lateral border is the pharyngeal ostium of the eustachian tube. It is lined with respiratory ciliated stratified squamous epithelium.

◆ Oropharynx – this extends downwards from the nasopharynx to the superior edge of the epiglottis. It contains the palatine tonsils with the anterior and posterior faucial pillars, and the bodies of the second and third cervical vertebrae. It is lined with stratified squamous epithelium.

◆ Hypopharynx – this extends from the superior edge of the epiglottis to the inferior edge of the cricoid cartilage. It lies posterior to the larynx, medial to both pyriform fossae and the inferior constrictor muscles, and anterior to the third to sixth cervical vertebrae. Inferiorly it opens into the oesophagus, and it is lined with stratified squamous epithelium.

Pharyngeal musculature (Figs 32 and 33)

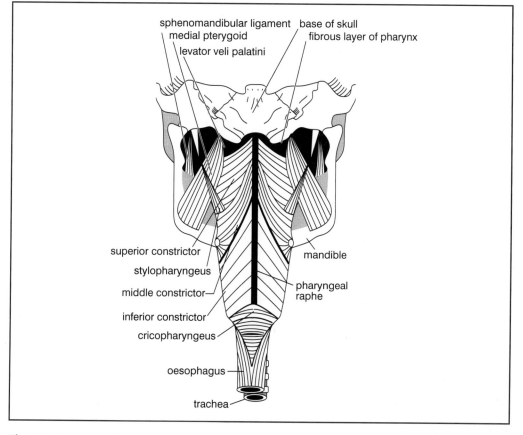

Fig. 32 Anatomy of the pharynx

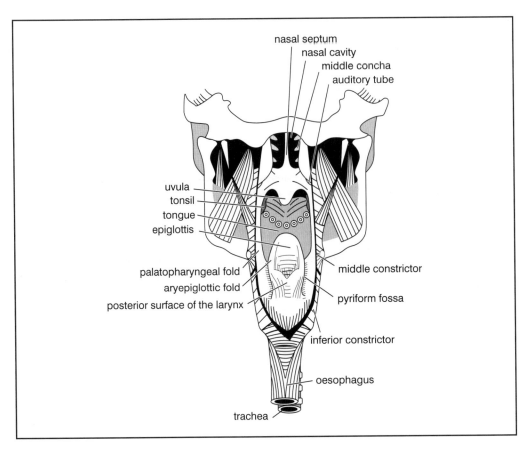

Fig. 33 Interior of the pharynx

The pharynx is surrounded by a circular muscle layer consisting of the superior, middle and inferior constrictor muscles. The inferior constrictor divides into the thyropharyngeus above and the cricopharyngeus below. The gap between them is known as 'Killian's dehiscence', and marks the point of herniation of a pharyngeal pouch. The pharynx is raised and lowered by three pairs of muscles:

◆ stylopharyngeus
◆ salpingopharyngeus
◆ palatopharyngeus.

Vascular supply

Branches of the external carotid artery – including the ascending pharyngeal artery, the ascending and descending palatine artery, and branches of the lingual, facial and maxillary arteries. Venous drainage is to the internal jugular vein.

Nerve supply

- Motor: glossopharyngeal, vagus, hypoglossal and facial nerves
- Sensory:
  - nasopharynx – maxillary division of trigeminal nerve
  - oropharynx – glossopharyngeal nerve
  - hypopharynx – vagus nerve

Snoring and sleep apnoea

Partial airway obstruction during sleep causes generation of noise and restriction in airflow with consequent apnoea (more than ten seconds without airflow).

Snoring

- This is the vibration of pharyngeal walls caused by turbulent airflow.
- It can be caused by obstruction anywhere in the airway (eg nasal septum, nasopharynx, soft palate, oropharynx, hypopharynx).
- Lack of tone of pharyngeal muscle wall may be a factor.
- Neck obesity also implicated.
- It is more common in older overweight men.
- It may lead to serious social consequences.

Sleep apnoea

- It is defined as more than 30 apnoeic episodes in seven hours of sleep or more than five per hour.
- It may lead to hypoxia and increased cardiovascular strain.
- It may lead to daytime somnolence.

Investigations

- Body mass index (BMI)
- Thyroid function tests (TFTs), chest X-ray (CXR), electrocardiogram (ECG)
- Epworth score to assess daytime somnolence
- Sleep study to identify sleep apnoea
- Müller's manoeuvre – inhalation with mouth and nose closed while a fibreoptic naso-endoscope views the oro- and hypopharynx. This identifies any areas of collapse
- Sleep nasoendoscopy

Treatment

- Often many causes for the apnoea
- Advice on lifestyle changes and weight loss
- Improvement of nasal airway through septoplasty or turbinate surgery
- Continuous positive airways pressure (CPAP) for severe obstructive sleep apnoea (OSA)

- Treatment of oropharyngeal obstruction by adenotonsillectomy/uvulopalatoplasty
- Moving of tongue base forward using mandibular positioning device during sleep
- Tracheostomy – only for very severe cases

Uvulopalatoplasty

- Usually involves tonsillectomy
- Excision of the uvula
- Can be performed with diathermy, cold steel or laser
- Newer techniques involve radiofrequency energy applied to soft palate to scar and stiffen
- Risks – pain, bleeding, failure, nasal regurgitation

Tonsillitis

This is thought to be caused by viral or bacterial infection:

- Bacterial – streptococci (β-haemolytic), staphylococci, pneumococci, *H. influenzae*, *E. coli.*
- Viral – rhinovirus, adenovirus, enterovirus, Epstein–Barr virus.
- Other infections – *Bacteroides fragilis, Corynebacterium diphtheriae, Treponema pallidum, Mycobacterium tuberculosis, Candida,* Vincent's spirillum without fuso-bacterium (Vincent's angina presents as an ulcerated swelling on one tonsil, with minimal pain symptoms and ipsilateral node swelling).

Tonsillitis may be non-infective – leukaemia, lymphoma.

Clinical features

- Pyrexia, malaise, lack of appetite
- Dysphagia
- Lymphadenopathy
- Odynophagia
- Trismus
- Swollen tonsils with or without exudate
- Otalgia (effect on glossopharyngeal nerve)

Management

- Analgesia
- Antibiotics (not amoxicillin as this may induce a maculopapular rash in infectious mononucleosis)
- Drainage of any peritonsillar abscess
- Antiseptic gargles
- Tonsillectomy if frequent recurrence

Glandular fever often presents with tonsillar exudate, although the Paul–Bunnell test may not be positive initially. Patients suspected of having glandular fever should be strongly advised to avoid contact sport for 2–3 months after infection as the virus may have caused hepatosplenomegaly.

Complications

◆ Peritonsillar abscess (quinsy)
◆ Retropharyngeal abscess
◆ Parapharyngeal abscess
◆ Acute otitis media
◆ Septicaemia
◆ Meningitis
◆ Glomerulonephritis/rheumatic fever (due to streptococcal illness)

Tonsillectomy

Indications

◆ Recurrent tonsillitis (at least five episodes per year for at least 2 years, or more than one quinsy)
◆ Sleep apnoea syndrome
◆ Suspected neoplasm
◆ Part of another procedure (eg uvulopharyngoplasty (UVPP))

Contraindications

◆ Acute infection
◆ Bleeding disorder
◆ Cleft palate

Procedure

A Boyle–Davis mouth gag is inserted, and the mouth is opened as wide as possible. The tonsils are removed using a variety of methods, eg cold-steel dissection, diathermy, laser, co-ablation or guillotine. It is important to achieve haemostasis at the end of the operation and to check the postnasal space for a clot. Haemorrhage is the most frequent complication, and it is thought to occur in 2–5% of cases. It generally occurs from the tonsillar artery or one of its branches. The bleeding can be:

◆ primary (within 24 hours of surgery)
◆ secondary (commonly 5–10 days postoperatively).

Recent research has suggested that the use of diathermy is associated with a higher secondary haemorrhage rate. Intractable bleeding may be treated with local application of an adrenaline pack, but it may necessitate a return to theatre and suturing of the anterior and posterior faucial pillars together over a swab.

Complications

- Haemorrhage
- Infection
- Tooth damage
- Temporomandibular joint (TMJ) dislocation
- Voice change
- Otalgia
- Trauma to soft palate/posterior pharyngeal wall

Oral carcinomas

- 90% are squamous cell carcinomas.
- Betel nut-chewing/smoking/alcohol are risk factors.
- Male:female ratio is 2:1.
- Commonest sites: the lateral border of the tongue and the floor of the mouth.
- 30% have second primaries present.

TNM staging for oral carcinomas

- T1   < 2 cm
- T2   2–4 cm
- T3   > 4 cm
- T4   extension to bone/muscle/skin

Clinical features

- Painful ulcer
- Halitosis
- Dysphagia
- Speech problems
- Neck lumps

Investigations

- CT/bone scan to illustrate bone invasion
- MRI for tongue tumours
- CXR
- Examination under anaesthetic (EUA) and biopsy

Management

- T1/2 – surgery or external beam/implant radiotherapy
- T3/4 – partial/total glossectomy

◆ Neck nodes – almost all cases require ipsilateral selective neck dissection or radiotherapy at least, and, because of lymphatic crossover, contralateral treatment should be considered
◆ Post-operative radiotherapy for large tumours/positive margins.

Swallowing

The mouth and pharynx are responsible for mastication and initiation of swallowing, which can be divided into three phases.

Phases of swallowing

◆ **Oral phase** – chewing and the digestive and lubricating action of saliva prepare the food bolus for swallowing. The bolus is then moved posteriorly by the tongue moving upwards and when the bolus reaches the base of the tongue the swallowing reflex is initiated.
◆ **Pharyngeal phase** – the nasopharynx and trachea are closed off by the action of the soft palate and vocal cords, respectively. The bolus travels downwards through the pyriform fossae by contraction of the constrictor muscles. It travels into the hypopharynx, where it stimulates the oesophageal orifice to open.
◆ **Oesophageal phase** – involuntary peristalsis of the oesophageal muscles propels the bolus through the oesophagus to the stomach.

The **swallowing reflex** is initiated by sensory impulses from the trigeminal, glossopharyngeal and vagus nerves. These impulses travel to the medulla oblongata, where efferent impulses are generated to the vagus, accessory and hypoglossal nerves. Swallowing may be affected by disorders of the vagus, glossopharyngeal or hypoglossal nerves.

Dysphagia

Dysphagia – difficulty in swallowing and eating.
Odynophagia – pain on swallowing.

Causes

◆ In the mouth:
  ● dental
  ● aphthous ulcers
  ● carcinoma
  ● anaemia
  ● systemic lupus erythematosus (SLE)
  ● Sjögren's syndrome
◆ In the oropharynx:
  ● tonsillitis
  ● carcinoma
  ● pharyngitis

- In the oesophagus:
  - inflammation
  - constriction
  - foreign body
- In the hypopharynx:
  - pharyngeal pouch
  - achalasia
  - carcinoma
  - neurological disease
  - foreign body

Assessment

- History
- Examination – mouth, oropharynx
- Endoscopy
- Barium swallow

Globus pharyngeus

This is the sensation of a lump, discomfort or foreign body in the throat with no obvious cause.

Possible aetiology

- Reflux
- Disorder of oesophageal/pharyngeal motility
- Psychological effects

Clinical features

- Often female patients, most commonly in their forties
- Ache rather than a sharp pain
- Tends to be constant rather than worse during swallowing

Management

- Barium swallow to exclude organic lesion
- Endoscopy if symptoms are suspicious
- pH measurement
- Trial of antireflux therapy
- Treatment of any psychological factors
- Reassurance

Tongue and taste

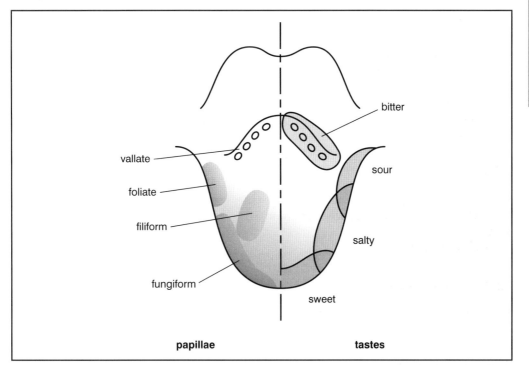

Fig. 34 Tongue with taste areas and papillae regions

Many foods are 'tasted' by the olfactory nerve, but the sensations of sweet, salty, bitter and sour are exclusive to the taste system. The various sensations are picked up on the tongue, as shown in Fig. 34, by the taste buds. These lie in the vallate papillae (in front of the sulcus) and fungiform papillae (peripherally), and saliva is required as a transport medium to facilitate tasting. The filiform papillae do not contain taste receptors. The sensory supply of the anterior two-thirds of the tongue comes from the lingual nerve, a branch of the trigeminal nerve, with taste supplied by the chorda tympani, a branch of the facial nerve. In the posterior two-thirds of the tongue, both taste and sensation are supplied by the glossopharyngeal nerve alone. The sulcus terminalis divides the tongue into the two sections. The inferior surface of the tongue has the frenum in the midline, with the lingual artery, nerve and vein present more laterally. The sublingual glands and submandibular ducts open here as well.

Muscles of the tongue

◆ Intrinsic – superior and inferior longitudinal, transverse, vertical (all supplied by hypoglossal nerve)
◆ Extrinsic – genioglossus, hyoglossus, styloglossus (all supplied by hypoglossal nerve), palatoglossus (supplied by cranial root of accessory nerve)

Lymphatic drainage

- Posterior one-third – to the deep cervical nodes
- Anterior two-thirds – via submandibular nodes to the deep cervical nodes
- Tip – via submental nodes

Nasopharyngeal carcinomas

- Squamous keratinising, squamous, non-keratinising, or undifferentiated.
- Epstein–Barr virus is a risk factor in combination with a genetic predisposition.
- A diet of salt-preserved fish, as seen in Hong Kong, predisposes.
- Mostly originate in the fossa of Rosenmüller.
- May cause facial nerve or eustachian tube involvement.

TNM staging of nasopharyngeal carcinomas

- T1   confined to nasopharynx
- T2   extending to soft tissue of oropharynx or nasal fossa
- T3   invading bone or sinuses
- T4   invading cranial fossae/hypopharynx/orbit/infratemporal fossa

Clinical features

- Neck lump
- Otalgia
- Epistaxis

Treatment

- Most tumours are treated with radiotherapy.
- Bilateral neck irradiation may also be indicated as prophylaxis against future neck metastases.
- Radical neck dissection for resistant/recurrent disease.

Angiofibroma

- Benign tumour consisting of fibrous and vascular tissue.
- Involves the sphenopalatine foramen.
- Epistaxis, bone erosion and nasal obstruction may be present.
- Surgical removal involves mid-facial degloving or craniofacial approach.
- Preoperative embolisation may assist removal of large tumours.

Oropharyngeal carcinomas

- 85% are squamous cell carcinomas:
  - male:female ratio 5:1
  - 30% have a second primary within ten years.

- 10% are non-Hodgkin's lymphoma – mostly palatine or lingual tonsil.
- 2% are minor salivary gland carcinomas – mostly from lateral wall, 50% adenoid cystic.
- 3% others.
- Leukoplakia is premalignant.
- Risk factors:
  - smoking (made worse by alcohol)
  - betel nut-chewing.

TNM staging of oropharyngeal carcinomas

- T1   < 2 cm
- T2   2–4 cm
- T3   > 4 cm
- T4   extending beyond oropharynx

Clinical features

- Neck lump
- Sore throat
- Odynophagia
- Muffled speech
- Trismus (pterygoid involvement)

Investigations

- MRI for definition of soft tissue involvement
- CXR and liver ultrasound
- Fine-needle aspiration cytology (FNAC) of any lump felt
- Panendoscopy
- Tonsil/tongue base biopsy

Management

- Squamous cell carcinoma/minor salivary gland carcinoma: T1–2 radiotherapy, T3–4 1–2-cm clearance margin required ± neo-adjuvant chemoradiotherapy
- Non-Hodgkin's lymphoma – CHOP/VAPEC-B chemotherapy regimen:
  - CHOP – cyclophosphamide; doxorubicin; Oncovin® (vincristine); prednisolone
  - VAPEC-B – vincristine; doxorubicin (originally known as Adriamycin®); prednisolone; etoposide; cyclophosphamide; bleomycin

Surgical clearance

Depends on the stage and site of involvement:

- Mandibulectomy

◆ Glossopharyngectomy
◆ Palatectomy
◆ Total larygopharyngo-oesophagectomy
◆ Reconstruction with radial forearm flap
◆ Selective/modified-radical/radical neck dissection.

Adjuvant radiotherapy may be required for positive margins. Swallowing rehabilitation and treatment for strictures may also be needed.

Hypopharyngeal carcinomas

◆ 90% are squamous cell carcinomas
◆ Older age group, more common in men than in women
◆ Three anatomical sites:
  ● postcricoid – 60%
  ● pyriform fossa – 30%
  ● posterior pharyngeal wall – 10%

TNM staging of hypopharyngeal carcinomas

◆ T1   one site and < 2 cm
◆ T2   more than one site, or 2–4 cm
◆ T3   > 4 cm, or fixation of hemilarynx
◆ T4   invasion of adjacent structures

Clinical features

◆ Neck lump
◆ Hoarseness
◆ Dysphagia
◆ Pneumonia

Investigations

◆ Full blood count (FBC)
◆ Barium swallow
◆ MRI
◆ CXR
◆ Panendoscopy/bronchoscopy

Management

◆ Radiotherapy for early tumours.
◆ Surgery for large tumours or metastases, which may involve lateral pharyngotomy or

total laryngopharyngectomy with reconstruction. Speech rehabilitation may be necessary. Removal of the thyroid requires hormone replacement.
◆ Combined therapy – surgery and adjuvant radiotherapy for large tumours or small margins.

INFRATEMPORAL FOSSA

Boundaries

◆ Medial – lateral pterygoid plate, pterygomaxillary fissure, superior constrictor of pharynx, tensor palati, levator veli palatini
◆ Lateral – ramus of the mandible
◆ Anterior – posterior surface of the maxilla, inferior orbital fissure
◆ Posterior – carotid sheath
◆ Roof – greater wing of sphenoid, squamous part of temporal bone

Contents

◆ Insertion of temporalis
◆ Maxillary artery and branches – the artery passes between the two heads of the lateral pterygoid to enter the pterygopalatine fossa. It has 15 branches, including the inferior alveolar, middle meningeal, sphenopalatine and infraorbital arteries
◆ Pterygoid venous plexus
◆ Mandibular nerve and branches – the nerve emerges from the skull through the foramen ovale. It has nine branches, including the nerves to medial and lateral pterygoid, lingual nerve, inferior alveolar nerve and auriculotemporal nerve
◆ Medial and lateral pterygoid muscles
◆ Otic ganglion
◆ Chorda tympani
◆ Posterior alveolar nerve

Muscles of the infratemporal fossa

Muscle	Origin	Insertion	Nerve supply	Action
Lateral pterygoid muscle	Upper head – infratemporal surface of the skull Lower head – lateral surface of the lateral pterygoid plate	Pterygoid fossa on mandibular head	Anterior division of mandibular nerve	Draws condyle forward, opens mouth
Medial pterygoid muscle	Deep head – medial surface of the lateral pterygoid plate Superficial head – tuberosity of maxilla, pyramidal process of the palatine bone	Inner surface of the angle of mandible	Mandibular nerve	Closes mouth, moves mandible to opposite side in chewing

Table 9 The pterygoid muscles

LARYNX AND TRACHEA

Anatomy of the larynx

The skeleton of the larynx consists of the thyroid, cricoid and arytenoid hyaline cartilages, the epiglottis (which is made up of fibrous cartilage) and fibroelastic accessory cartilage. Calcification begins at puberty and occurs earlier in boys – calcifications may be confused with foreign bodies.

Laryngeal compartments

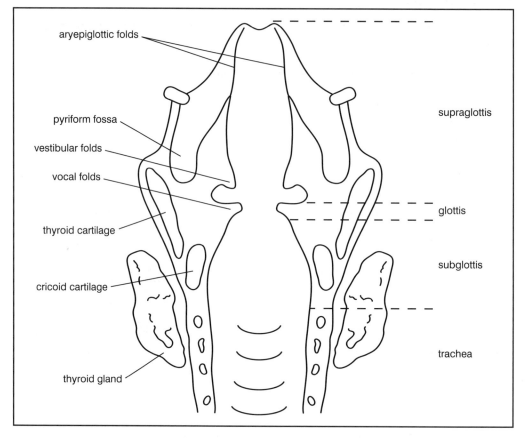

Fig. 35 Laryngeal compartments

◆ Supraglottis:
  ● laryngeal surface of epiglottis
  ● aryepiglottic fold
  ● vestibular folds
  ● ventricle as far as the superior surface of the vocal folds
◆ Glottis – vocal folds and 1 cm inferiorly
◆ Subglottis – down to lower border of the cricoid cartilage

Vocal cords

The vocal cords are made up of layers (Fig. 36). From most superficial to deep these are:

◆ stratified squamous epithelium
◆ Reinke's space
◆ vocal ligament
◆ thyroarytenoid/vocalis muscle.

Muscles that control the larynx

Internal muscles and one external muscle (cricothyroid) (Fig. 37) act to control the larynx as follows:

◆ Cord abduction – posterior cricoarytenoid muscle.
◆ Cord adduction:
  ● lateral cricoarytenoid muscle
  ● transverse arytenoid muscle
  ● thyroarytenoid muscle.
◆ Tension of the vocal folds:
  ● cricothyroid muscle
  ● thyroarytenoid muscle.

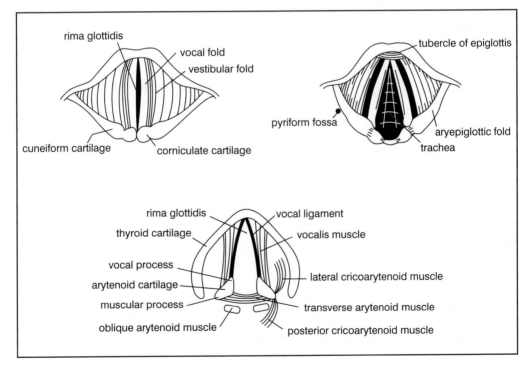

Fig. 36 Vocal cords and the epiglottis from above

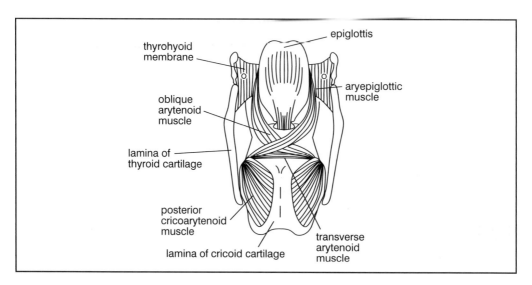

Fig. 37 Cartilages and muscles of larynx

Nerve supply

This is by the vagus nerve, which divides into laryngeal nerves as follows:

- Superior laryngeal nerve (SLN):
  - sensory internal branch supplies interior of larynx to glottis
  - motor external branch supplies cricothyroid muscle.
- Recurrent laryngeal nerve (RLN) – sensory supply to laryngeal mucosa inferior to glottis.

Motor supply to internal laryngeal musculature

The left RLN loops around the aortic arch and travels in the groove between the trachea and oesophagus; the right RLN passes under the subclavian artery and then upwards in the tracheo-oesophageal groove. Both enter the larynx at the inferior cornu of the thyroid cartilage.

Relations

The relations of the SLN, RLN and the thyroid arteries are as follows:

- Superior thyroid artery – branch of external carotid, arches inferiorly to attain upper pole of the thyroid gland. Early in its path it lies close to the external branch of the SLN.
- Inferior thyroid artery – from the thyrocervical trunk, it bends medially at C6, and enters the lower pole of thyroid gland, where it lies close to the RLN on either side. In 25% the RLN lies anterior to the artery, in 35% posterior to the artery, and in 35% between the branches of the artery.

Anatomy of the trachea

The trachea is 10 cm in length, extending from the level of C6 downwards. It is made of C-shaped hyaline cartilage rings, trachealis muscle posteriorly and a fibroelastic membrane.

Relations

- Anteriorly – inferior thyroid vein, anterior jugular venous arch, thyroid ima artery, thyroid isthmus
- Posteriorly – oesophagus, RLN
- Laterally – carotid sheath, thyroid lobes

Blood supply

Inferior thyroid artery.

Nerve supply

- Parasympathetic – vagus and recurrent laryngeal nerves
- Sympathetic – upper ganglia of the sympathetic trunk

Laryngeal carcinomas

- Mostly squamous cell carcinomas
- Male:female ratio 5:1
- Smoking is the main risk factor
- Synchronous tumours in up to 5%
- Sites – supraglottic/glottis/subglottis

TNM staging of laryngeal carcinomas

- T1   only one site
- T2   extension to another site
- T3   fixed vocal cord or postcricoid invasion
- T4   extension beyond larynx

Clinical features

- Hoarseness
- Dysphagia/odynophagia
- Dyspnoea

Investigations

- CXR
- FBC/liver function tests (LFTs)
- MRI/CT (including chest and abdomen)
- Panendoscopy and EUA of neck

Management

- T1–2 – radiotherapy or partial laryngectomy
- T3 – total laryngectomy ± postoperative radiotherapy
- T4 – total laryngectomy with neck dissection
- Voice restoration procedure and speech therapy
- Thyroid/parathyroid hormone supplementation if necessary

Laryngectomy

- Performed for carcinoma, in conjunction with a voice restoration procedure and radiotherapy if appropriate.
- Appropriate preoperative patient counselling is vital.

Types

- Cordectomy – endoscopic or open, also used for benign tumours.
- Hemilaryngectomy – this is for tumours confined to vocal fold; half thyroid and cricoid cartilage removed, strap muscle fashioned into new vocal cord.
- Supraglottic laryngectomy – this is the joining of the glottis to the base of the tongue, vocal cords intact.
- Supracricoid partial laryngectomy – this may involve removal of vocal folds/thyroid cartilage/epiglottis and one arytenoid cartilage.
- Total laryngectomy – this is for curative treatment; involves removal of thyroid/hyoid and cricoid cartilages, proximal trachea and thyroid gland. A tracheostome with speech valve is required.

Vocal pathology

Voice is assessed ideally by videolaryngostroboscopy and analysis of voice patterns, conducted in a specialist voice clinic with speech and language therapy and ENT input. Vocal pathology can be divided into the following:

- hyperfunctional, eg muscle tension dysphonia, nodules, polyps, haemorrhage, ulcers
- psychogenic
- structural abnormalities, eg web, cleft palate, sulcus vocalis, trauma, presbylarynx
- neurogenic, eg parkinsonism, spasmodic dysphonia, multiple sclerosis
- endocrinological, eg thyrotoxicosis, drug effects
- neoplasia

- disease affecting the larynx, eg papillomatosis, reflux
- inflammatory conditions, eg autoimmune disease, fungal infection.

Treatment

- Advice about vocal hygiene
- Speech and language therapy
- Antacid treatments
- Operative excision
- Botulinum toxin injection

Stridor

Stridor is a bovine-like inspiratory noise associated with laryngeal obstruction, more common in children.

Causes

- Adults:
  - extraluminal
  - neurological
  - iatrogenic (eg after thyroidectomy)
  - trauma
  - mural
  - angioneurotic oedema
  - granuloma
  - malignancy
  - laryngomalacia
  - luminal
  - TB
  - foreign body
- Children:
  - extraluminal
  - trauma
  - mediastinal tumour
  - anomalous blood vessels
  - vagal or laryngeal nerve paralysis
  - mural
  - angioneurotic oedema
  - laryngeal web
  - subglottic stenosis
  - laryngotracheobronchitis
  - laryngeal papillomatosis
  - acute laryngitis
  - acute epiglottitis

Management

- Remove false teeth and secretions.
- In emergency – endotracheal tube, cricothyroidotomy, jet insufflation.
- If time – laryngoscopy, adrenaline nebulisers, tracheostomy if longer-term intubation is needed.

Tracheostomy

Indications

- Relief of airway obstruction – congenital, traumatic, infection, tumour, bilateral cord paralysis, foreign body, sleep apnoea syndrome.
- Protection of the tracheobronchial tree – neurological disease (eg multiple sclerosis), trauma, coma, head and neck surgery.
- Treatment of respiratory insufficiency – chest injury, pulmonary disease.

Procedure

1 Give general anaesthesia in emergency (local anaesthetic)
2 Extend the patient's head.
3 Make a transverse skin incision 2 cm below cricoid cartilage (midline vertical incision in emergency).
4 Separate the strap muscles.
5 Retract or divide the thyroid isthmus.
6 Cut the disc from the 2nd/3rd tracheal rings.
7 Aspirate the trachea and insert the tube.
8 Close the skin edges.

Complications

- Early – aspiration, asphyxia, haemorrhage, obstruction, emphysema, pneumothorax, cricoid cartilage injury.
- Late – cellulitis, subglottic stenosis, vocal cord palsy, tracheocutaneous or tracheo-oesophageal fistula, displacement of tube, atelectasis, tracheomalacia, dysphagia, tracheal stenosis, difficult decannulation.

Note: Tracheostomy for relief of airway obstruction due to carcinoma is associated with a high rate of stomal recurrence; some feel that emergency laryngectomy should be carried out instead.

THYROID GLAND

Anatomy

The thyroid gland is surrounded by its own capsule and pretracheal fascia. Each lobe has three surfaces: lateral, medial and posterior.

Relations

- Lateral surface – sternothyroid, sternocleidomastoid, sternohyoid
- Medial surface – external laryngeal nerve, recurrent laryngeal nerve, larynx, pharynx, oesophagus, trachea
- Posterior surface – parathyroid glands, carotid sheath and contents, inferior thyroid artery, thoracic duct (on the left side only)

Blood supply

- Superior and inferior thyroid arteries

Venous drainage:

- superior thyroid vein to internal jugular or facial vein
- middle thyroid vein to internal jugular vein
- inferior thyroid vein via plexus to brachiocephalic veins

Lymphatic drainage

- Upper pole to anterior-superior group of deep cervical nodes
- Lower pole to posterior-inferior group of deep cervical nodes

The thyroid gland first appears at the site of the foramen caecum in the floor of the pharynx and descends to reach its final position by the seventh week of gestation. It remains connected to the tongue by the thyroglossal duct, and so thyroglossal cysts can be found along this path of descent. They are cystic remains of the thyroglossal duct. Accessory thyroid tissue can be found in the tongue, near the hyoid bone, deep to sternocleidomastoid and in the superior mediastinum.

Physiology

The thyroid produces:

- thyroxine (T_4)
- tri-iodothyronine (T_3)
- calcitonin.

Thyroxine and T_3 are synthesised in the colloid of the thyroid gland by the iodination of tyrosine molecules bound to thyroglobulin. Iodine (I^-) is absorbed from plasma and converted to iodine (I_2) by thyroid peroxidase in the follicular cells. Most of the thyroxine and T_3 circulate in plasma bound to proteins, including thyroxine-binding globulin (TBG), thyroxine-binding pre-albumin (TBPA) and albumin. T_3 is more potent than thyroxine and so thyroxine is converted to T_3 by de-iodination. The thyroid hormones act by entering the cell and attaching to nuclear receptors. These bind to DNA, which leads to increased production of mRNA and increased expression of certain genes.

Thyroid function is controlled by a negative feedback mechanism, with increased levels of thyroxine and T_3 detected by the hypothalamus and anterior pituitary. The hypothalamus releases thyroid-releasing hormone (TRH), which travels through the portal system of blood vessels to reach the anterior pituitary. Thyroid-stimulating hormone (TSH), a glycoprotein, travels in the bloodstream to act on the thyroid gland. It acts by binding to receptors on the cell membrane and causing increased c-AMP production within the cell.

Thyroid hormones stimulate oxygen consumption in most of the body's cells and increase the sensitivity of β-receptors to catecholamines. Their actions include:

◆ increased protein catabolism
◆ increased fat mobilisation and degradation
◆ increased gluconeogenesis, glycogenolysis and glucose absorption from the gut
◆ normal development of the central nervous system
◆ regulation of gut mobility and hair and skin development.

From the above, the features of hyperthyroidism, cretinism and myxoedema can be explained.

Hyperthyroidism (thyrotoxicosis)

Causes

◆ Graves' disease
◆ Solitary toxic nodule
◆ Toxic multinodular goitre
◆ Overdoes of thyroxine
◆ Thyroid carcinoma
◆ Iodine therapy
◆ Hyperfunctioning ovarian teratoma

Clinical features

◆ Heat intolerance
◆ Low blood cholesterol
◆ Anxiety and irritability
◆ Diarrhoea
◆ Muscle wasting
◆ Weight loss

- Tremor
- Tachycardia and arrhythmias
- Menstrual irregularities

Treatment

- Medical
- Radioactive iodine
- Surgical

Hypothyroidism

Causes

- Autoimmune thyroiditis (Hashimoto's, atrophic thyroiditis)
- Iodine deficiency
- Post-irradiation
- Tumour infiltration
- Antithyroid drugs
- Hypopituitarism

Clinical features

- Cold intolerance
- Increased blood cholesterol
- Sluggish mental activity
- Menstrual irregularities
- Weight increase
- Tiredness
- Bradycardia
- Cretinism, if occurring prenatally

Treatment

- Thyroxine

Thyroid swelling

Causes

- Solitary nodule – multinodular goitre, adenoma, carcinoma, haemorrhage into a cyst
- Diffuse swelling – multinodular goitre, Hashimoto's thyroiditis, Graves' disease, carcinoma

Investigations

- TFTs (T_3, T_4, TSH)
- TRH test

- Ultrasound
- Fine-needle aspiration (FNA)
- Thyroid autoantibodies (eg in Hashimoto's thyroiditis)

Thyroid tumours

- Benign:
  - **Adenomas** – these are common and often multiple. Can be solid of filled with colloid and can cause hyperthyroidism.
- Malignant:
  - **Papillary adenocarcinoma** (70% of tumours) – the commonest malignant thyroid cancer, seen in younger patients with a history of irradiation to the neck. Multifocal disease can be seen and frequently spreads to cervical lymph nodes. Histological appearance includes the presence of 'Orphan Annie' nuclei (pale, empty-looking). Most tumours are TSH-dependent. The treatment of papillary carcinoma is controversial. Treatment can consist of total thyroidectomy with thyroxine (to prevent TSH excretion) or unilateral lobectomy with thyroxine. Ten-year survival is 90%.
  - **Follicular carcinoma** (20% of thyroid tumours) – a unifocal tumour of the thyroid, composed of malignant glandular tissue. Can spread via the bloodstream in addition to lymph nodes. Treated by total thyroidectomy. Ten-year survival is 85%.
  - **Anaplastic carcinoma** (< 5% of thyroid tumours) – this is seen in older patients and has the worst prognosis. Rapidly metastasises to lymph nodes and also spreads directly to adjacent tissues. Treatment consists of debulking surgery and external beam radiotherapy. Five-year survival is poor.
  - **Medullary carcinoma** (5% of thyroid tumours) – a tumour of C cells (calcitonin-secreting cells). Familial tendency, therefore screen for multiple endocrine neoplasia (MEN) syndromes. These tumours can be multifocal and spread via blood and to lymph nodes. The treatment consists of total thyroidectomy.

Thyroidectomy

Indications

- Overactivity, where other treatments have failed
- Cosmesis
- Compression
- Carcinoma

Preoperative preparation

Patients should be rendered euthyroid by means of carbimazole and β blockers, otherwise a thyroid crisis may be precipitated during the operation.

Procedure

The neck is extended and a horizontal incision is made through skin, subcutaneous fat and platysma. Investing fascia and connective tissue is incised vertically. Strap muscles are divided if necessary. The thyroid lobe is mobilised. The superior thyroid artery is tied off close to the gland to avoid the external laryngeal nerve. The inferior artery is tied off laterally far away from the gland to avoid the RLN. Some tie off the inferior thyroid artery in continuity to avoid transecting the laryngeal nerve.

In a subtotal thyroidectomy it is acceptable to leave a sliver of gland laterally in front of the parathyroids and RLN. In a total thyroidectomy the thyroid must be dissected free from those structures. The isthmus is dissected with care, avoiding damage to the trachea, and oversewn in a lobectomy. Closure is in layers, usually with a suction drain and clips to skin.

Complications

- Post-operative bleeding
- SLN/RLN damage
- Temporary or permanent hypocalcaemia (due to parathyroid damage)

PARATHYROID GLANDS

Anatomy

There are usually four glands, located outside or inside the pretracheal fascia. The superior glands lie at the level of the first tracheal ring, while the inferior glands lie closely applied to the inferior pole of the thyroid below the inferior thyroid artery. However, the position of the lower parathyroids can be much lower, for example in the superior mediastinum. They are supplied by the inferior thyroid artery and are approached operatively as for the thyroid gland.

Embryonic origin

- Superior parathyroids – fourth pharyngeal pouch
- Inferior parathyroids – third pharyngeal pouch

Physiology

The normal serum calcium concentration is 2.2–2.6 mmol/l. Only 1% of the total body calcium is not contained in bone. A patient's serum calcium level can be altered by the serum albumin level, because 40% of calcium in the blood is transported bound to albumin. The functions of calcium include:

- blood clotting
- muscle contraction
- nerve conduction
- co-factor in many enzyme reactions
- constituent of bone and teeth

- maintenance of normal permeability of cell membrane
- maintenance of excitability of nerve and muscle.

The hormones involved in calcium balance are:

- Parathyroid hormone (PTH) – increases resorption and decreases excretion of calcium, and increases phosphate excretion in urine.
- Vitamin D – increases resorption of calcium from the gut, decreases calcium excretion in urine and inhibits parathyroid hormone gene transcription.
- Calcitonin – reduces calcium resorption from bone and reduces calcium resorption from gut.

Hyperparathyroidism

- Primary – this is usually due to single or multiple parathyroid adenomas or, rarely, carcinoma or primary parathyroid hyperplasia.
- Secondary – this is in response to low serum calcium (eg in renal failure), so serum PTH levels are raised while serum calcium is low or normal.
- Tertiary – this occurs after long-standing secondary hyperparathyroidism; the parathyroids become hyperplastic after long-term stimulation. It is most often seen in chronic renal failure. Both PTH and serum calcium levels are raised.

Clinical features

- Renal stones
- Bone pain, osteoclasts, pepper-pot skull and phalangeal subperiosteal erosions
- Depression
- Abdominal pain, peptic ulcer disease, acute pancreatitis and constipation
- Hypertension
- Hypercalcaemic crisis

Hypoparathyroidism

In surgical practice, hypoparathyroidism and hypocalcaemia are most often seen post-operatively (eg after thyroidectomy, parathyroidectomy or radical neck surgery) However, other causes include:

- acute pancreatitis
- chronic renal failure
- massive transfusion
- vitamin D deficiency.

Clinical features

- Paraesthesia
- Tetany

◆ Circumoral numbness
◆ Chvostek's sign – twitching of facial muscles when tapping the facial nerve
◆ Trousseau's sign – spasm of fingers and wrist when a sphygmomanometer is inflated around the arm for three minutes
◆ Dystonia
◆ Psychosis
◆ Convulsions

Treatment

◆ 10 ml iv calcium gluconate over five minutes
◆ 40 ml iv calcium gluconate over 24 hours
◆ Vitamin D derivates
◆ Oral calcium supplements
◆ Monitor serum calcium levels closely

SALIVARY GLANDS

Parotid gland

The parotid gland is situated in the space between the mastoid process, styloid process and ramus of the mandible. It has a surrounding layer of investing fascia, the parotid sheath. It is mainly a serous gland, with a few mucous acini. It has an upper pole and a lower pole, and lateral, anterior and deep surfaces.

Relations

◆ Anterior – masseter, medial pterygoid, stylomandibular ligament, superficial temporal and maxillary artery, facial nerve
◆ Deep surface – sternocleidomastoid, posterior belly of digastric, external carotid artery, mastoid process, styloid process with attached muscles and ligaments
◆ Within the gland – facial nerve (superficial), retromandibular vein, external carotid artery, auriculotemporal nerve (deep)

The parotid duct runs across the masseter and pierces the buccinator and drains opposite the second upper molar tooth.

Blood supply

Branches from the external carotid artery; venous drainage via the retromandibular vein.

Lymphatic drainage

This is to the deep cervical nodes.

Nerve supply

◆ Parasympathetic – secretomotor fibres; reach the parotid gland via the otic ganglion by 'hitch-hiking' along three nerves
◆ Sympathetic – vasoconstrictors from the superior cervical ganglion, the fibres travel via the external carotid artery plexus
◆ Sensory – auriculotemporal nerve

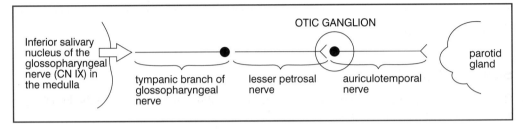

Fig. 38 Nerve supply of the parotid gland

Submandibular gland

The submandibular gland is divided into deep and superficial parts by the posterior border of mylohyoid. It is a mixed salivary gland, secreting mucous and serous saliva. The submandibular duct emerges from the superficial part of the gland. It enters the floor of the mouth next to the frenum. In its course it runs between the mylohyoid and hyoglossus muscles.

Relations of the superficial part of the submandibular gland

◆ Lateral – submandibular fossa of mandible, medial pterygoid, facial artery
◆ Inferior – skin, platysma, facial vein, cervical branch of the facial nerve
◆ Medial – mylohyoid muscle, hyoglossus muscle, lingual nerve (superior to deep part of gland), submandibular ganglion, hypoglossal nerve (inferior to deep part of gland), deep lingual vein, submandibular duct (inferior to deep part of gland)

Blood supply

Facial artery and vein.

Lymph drainage

Submandibular lymph nodes.

Nerve supply

◆ Parasympathetic – secretomotor fibres; reach the submandibular gland via the submandibular ganglion by 'hitch-hiking' along two nerves
◆ Sympathetic – vasoconstrictor from the plexus around the facial artery

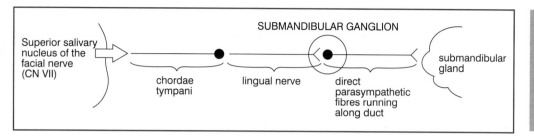

Fig. 39 Nerve supply of the submandibular gland

Sublingual gland

This is a mucus-secreting gland, which lies in front of the anterior border of the hyoglossus and medial to the genioglossus.

Relations

- Lateral – sublingual fossa of the mandible
- Medial – genioglossus
- Posterior – stylomandibular ligament, submandibular gland
- Anterior – opposite glands meet anteriorly
- Inferior – mylohyoid
- Superior – forms the sublingual fold of mucosa in the floor of the mouth

Blood supply

Lingual artery.

Nerve supply

Submandibular ganglion.

Salivary gland neoplasms

These can be divided into benign and malignant neoplasms. Furthermore, malignant tumours can be primary or secondary tumours.

- 80% of all salivary gland tumours occur in the parotid gland.
- 80% of all parotid tumours are benign – 80% of these are pleomorphic adenomas.
- 33% of tumours arising in the submandibular gland are malignant.
- 50% of tumours arising in the minor salivary glands are malignant.

Classification

- Benign tumours:
  - Pleomorphic adenomas – these present as a painless, enlarging smooth mass. Peak incidence is in fifth decade; equal male:female incidence. They have a pseudo-capsule and arise from myoepithelial cells and intercalated duct cells
  - Adenolymphoma (Warthin's tumour) – these are seen mainly in men (seven times more common than in women) aged 60–70 years. They are thought to arise from lymph nodes; 10% have bilateral tumours, but rarely at the same time
  - Myoepithelioma
  - Oncocytic adenoma
  - Ductal papilloma
  - Papillary cystadenoma
- Malignant tumours:
  - Adenoid cystic carcinoma – a slow-growing tumour which often spreads along nerve sheaths. The commonest malignant tumour of the salivary glands, it occurs more frequently in minor rather than major salivary glands. Patients may present with facial pain and facial nerve palsy. Tumours do not metastasise early and lymph node metastasis is uncommon. It occurs equally in men and women.
  - Adenocarcinoma – these make up 3% of parotid tumours and 10% of submandibular and minor salivary gland tumours
  - Carcinoma in pleomorphic adenoma
  - Squamous cell carcinoma
  - Undifferentiated carcinoma
- Tumours of variable malignancy:
  - Mucoepidermoid carcinoma – arise mainly in the parotid gland. They can behave in a benign or malignant fashion depending on degree of differentiation. Undifferentiated tumours metastasise early and carry a poor prognosis. They are the commonest salivary neoplasms in children
  - Acinic cell carcinoma
- Non-epithelial tumours:
  - Lymphangioma
  - Neurofibroma
  - Lymphoma
  - Haemangioma

Staging of malignant parotid gland tumours

- T0   no clinical evidence of tumour
- T1   < 2 cm diameter, without extraparenchymal extension
- T2   2–4 cm diameter, without extraparenchymal extension
- T3   4–6 cm diameter, and/or extraparenchymal extension
- T4   base of skull, seventh nerve involvement and/or > 6 cm

---

A parotid lump with involvement of the facial nerve (ie facial palsy) is highly suggestive of malignancy.

Investigations

♦ CT scan – this helps to assess relation of tumours to anatomical structures (eg facial nerve).
♦ FNA – this is a controversial issue; current guidelines recommend FNA at the first presentation and examination of the aspirate by an experienced pathologist.

Management of parotid gland tumours

The aim is to resect the tumour with a margin of macroscopically normal tissue, with preservation to the facial nerve. This is known as a 'formal conservative parotidectomy'. If the patient has a preoperative facial nerve palsy, a total parotidectomy is undertaken. Primary grafting of the facial nerve may be considered, but a frozen section of the facial nerve must be examined to ensure that the resection margins of the nerve are clear. Post-operative radiotherapy is indicated in certain cases:

♦ incomplete removal of pleomorphic adenoma or rupture at the time of removal
♦ if there is any doubt regarding resection margins
♦ if there is evidence of extracapsular spread
♦ high-grade tumours with high risk of local recurrence
♦ recurrent disease.

T1 and T2 tumours and pleomorphic adenomas removed with clear resection margins do not require post-operative radiotherapy.

Complications of a superficial parotidectomy

♦ Postoperative haemorrhage
♦ Sensory loss
♦ Salivary fistula
♦ Facial nerve palsy
♦ Frey's syndrome – gustatory sweating

Non-neoplastic infectious salivary gland disease

Acute sialoadenitis

♦ Viral:
  ● Mumps – this infection by paramyxovirus usually affects children aged 4–10 years; it is characterised by bilateral parotid swelling, malaise and trismus; it can also lead to orchitis, pancreatitis, nephritis, encephalitis, cochleitis and meningitis; usually self-limiting
  ● Coxsackievirus
  ● HIV
  ● Echovirus
♦ Bacterial:
  ● Usually staphylococcal infection, leading to pain, tenderness and discharge form the duct. It is most commonly seen in dehydrated and immunocompromised individuals. Treatment consists of systemic antibiotics and rehydration

Chronic recurrent sialoadenitis

This is a recurrent, slightly painful enlargement of the gland. It is due to impaired homoeostasis of salivary flow. Treatment consists of sialogogues, massage and hydration, or sialoadenectomy in refractory cases.

Granulomatous sialoadenitis

- Sarcoidosis
- TB
- Syphilis
- HIV

Non-neoplastic non-infectious salivary gland disease

Sialolithiasis

- Stones in the salivary glands lead to pain and swelling, worse at mealtimes.
- These are most commonly seen in middle-aged men.
- 80% of stones affect the submandibular gland; 65% of submandibular gland stones are radio-opaque, whereas 65% of parotid stones are radiolucent.
- Stones can be removed transorally.
- Sometimes submandibular gland resection must be undertaken.

Inflammatory conditions

- Sjögren's syndrome – this is an autoimmune disease defined by periductal lymphocytes in multiple organs. Around 40% of patients have salivary gland involvement and one in six patients will develop lymphoma. It is classified into:
  - primary Sjögren's syndrome (sicca complex) – identified by xerostomia, xeroph-thalmia and no connective tissue abnormality
  - secondary Sjögren's syndrome – comprises xerostomia, xerophthalmia and a connective tissue disorder, most commonly rheumatoid arthritis.
- Benign lymphoepithelial lesion – a mass of lymphoid tissue within a salivary gland containing scattered foci of epithelial cells of ductal origin. It is associated with HIV infection. The incidence of lymphoma arising from this condition is 10%.

Pseudoparotomegaly

The following may be confused with sialomegaly:

- winged mandible
- mandibular tumours
- dental cysts
- branchial cyst
- hypertrophic masseter
- neuroma of the facial nerve

- preauricular lymph node
- lipoma
- sebaceous cyst.

Drug-induced sialomegaly

- Oral contraceptive pill
- Thiouracil
- Co-proxamol
- Isoprenaline
- Phenylbutazone

Metabolic causes of sialomegaly

- Diabetes
- Myxoedema
- Cushing's disease
- Cirrhosis
- Gout
- Alcoholism
- Bulimia

Sialectasis

This is a disease of unknown origin recognised by progressive destruction of the alveoli and parenchyma of the gland with duct stenosis and cyst formation. Calculi may be found in the main ducts and patients often give a history of swelling exacerbated by eating.

During the clinical examination all the major salivary glands must be examined bimanually. Facial nerve palsy can be an indication of malignancy. Examination of the pharynx may show a lesion in the deep lobe of the parotid pushing the tonsil medially. In addition, a full ENT and general examination must be done. Investigations include erythrocyte sedimentation rate (ESR), FBC, rheumatoid factor, antinuclear factor, electrophoresis, anti-Ro and soluble liver antigen (SLA) antibodies, TFTs, blood glucose, routine LFTs, urate, plain film (submandibular calculus), sialogram (duct stenosis, calculi, sialectasis), CT/MRI (if neoplastic disease is suspected).

Biopsy: incisional or Trucut biopsy should not be performed due to the risk of seeding tumours; FNA may be useful. Sublabial biopsy is the investigation of choice in patients with suspected Sjögren's syndrome.

FACIAL NERVE

Anatomy

◆ Origin – junction of the pons and medulla.
◆ Components:
  ● motor root – special sensory (taste)
  ● parasympathetic – somatic sensory.
◆ During its course, the facial nerve traverses the following:
  ● posterior cranial fossa
  ● internal acoustic meatus
  ● facial canal in the temporal bone
  ● stylomastoid foramen
  ● parotid gland.
◆ The external marker of the main trunk of the facial nerve is the tragal pointer, 1 cm anterior and 2 cm inferior to the tragal cartilage.
◆ Facial nerve branches are given in Table 10.

Branches	Type of nerve	Structure supplied
Posterior auricular	Motor	Posterior belly of digastric, stylohyoid
Temporal	Motor	Muscles of facial expression
Zygomatic	Motor	Muscles of facial expression
Buccal	Motor	Muscles of facial expression
Mandibular	Motor	Muscles of facial expression
Cervical	Motor	Muscles of facial expression, platysma
Stapedius	Motor	Stapedius
Greater petrosal nerve	Parasympathetic secretomotor	Lacrimal gland (via synapse in the pterygopalatine ganglion)
Chorda tympani	Parasympathetic secretomotor	Submandibular and sublingual gland (via synapse in the submandibular ganglion
	Taste (joins the lingual nerve to supply the tongue)	Anterior two-thirds of the tongue
Fibres from the geniculate ganglion*	Somatic sensory	Area of skin around the external auditory meatus

*The sensory ganglion of the facial nerve is known as the geniculate ganglion and is located at the medial wall of the middle ear.

Table 10 Branches of the facial nerve

Muscles of facial expression

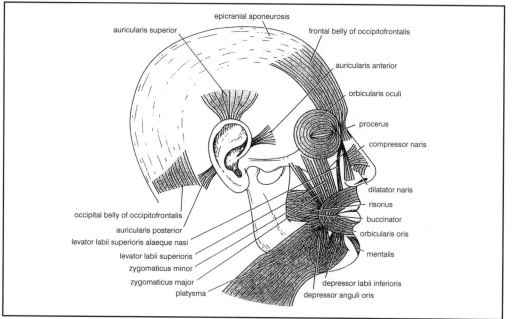

Fig. 40 Muscles of facial expression

The muscles are derived from the mesoderm of the second pharyngeal arch and are members of the panniculus carnosus.

Facial nerve palsy

◆ Lower motor neurone lesions – forehead involved
◆ Upper motor neurone lesions – forehead spared due to contralateral supply to lower motor neurone

The facial nerve has communications with many of the other cranial nerves, notably V, VIII, XI and X. This explains the referred pain in other areas of the face and neck associated with facial nerve disease.

Injury to any nerve may be classified as follows:

◆ Neuropraxia – complete absence of function without interruption of the nerve.
◆ Axonotmesis – damage to axon but nerve sheath still intact.
◆ Neurotmesis – damage to axon and also to surrounding tissue.
◆ Transection – complete division of the nerve.

Injury to the facial nerve may be graded according to the House–Brackmann grading system (see overleaf).

House–Brackmann grading system

I – Normal facial function
II – Slight weakness, normal symmetry and tone. Complete eye closure and forehead movement with effort, mouth slightly weak
III – Small difference between the two sides at rest. Complete eye closure with effort, slight to moderate forehead movement, mouth slightly weak
IV – Obvious weakness and disfiguring asymmetry. No forehead movement, incomplete eye closure and mouth asymmetrical
V – Only barely perceptible motion, asymmetrical at rest. No forehead movement, incomplete eye closure and slight mouth movement
VI – No movement

There may be other features, such as spasm:

◆ Synkinesis – movement of groups of muscles that do not usually contract together.
◆ Hemifacial spasm – an intermittent spasm of some or all of the facial muscles.
◆ Facial myokymia – multiple fine facial movements.
◆ Blepharospasm – involuntary spasmodic eye closure, which may be relieved by botulinum A toxin injection.
◆ Crocodile tears – lacrimation with eating, caused when regenerating motor nerve fibres connect to the greater petrosal nerve.

Causes of facial nerve palsy

◆ Bell's palsy (55%) – it is thought to be a virally induced lower motor neurone palsy, and it is a diagnosis of exclusion.
◆ Trauma (19%) – may be iatrogenic.
◆ Ramsay Hunt syndrome (7%) – herpes zoster virus causes facial palsy, and vesicles are often visible in the external ear canal and on the tympanic membrane.
◆ Tumour (6%) – the nerve may be affected due to direct pressure, invasion or growth in the nerve itself.
◆ Infection (4%) – otitis externa (acute, chronic or malignant (see page 39)) may cause facial nerve palsy, especially in the case of a dehiscence in the facial nerve canal.
◆ Other causes – these include multiple sclerosis, cerebrovascular accidents, myasthenia gravis and sarcoidosis.

Treatment

This should include eye protection and artificial tears. It may be necessary to aid eye closure by weighting the eyelid. Specific treatment may be necessary:

◆ Bell's palsy – this may require a course of high-dose steroids.
◆ Ramsay Hunt syndrome – aciclovir is often given and may shorten the duration of the palsy.

◆ Trauma – complete palsy immediately after trauma is an indication for exploration and attempted repair of the facial nerve.
◆ Tumour – sacrifice of the facial nerve may be necessary.
◆ Infection – palsy secondary to chronic otitis media indicates the need for mastoid exploration.

TRIGEMINAL NERVE

See Fig. 41 for the sensory supply of the face by the branches of the trigeminal nerve.

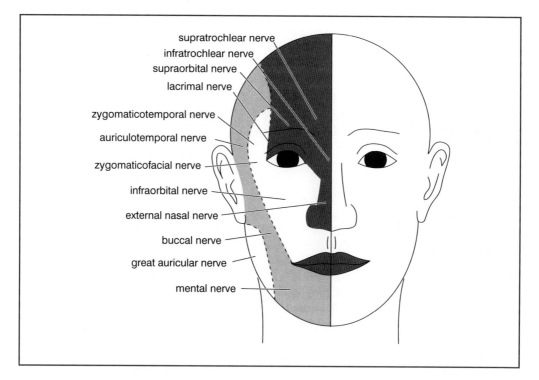

Fig. 41 Nerve supply to face

FOREIGN BODIES IN THE PHARYNX/LARYNX/OESOPHAGUS

Common objects

◆ Fish or meat bones
◆ Food bolus
◆ Coin
◆ Nuts or seeds
◆ Small toy parts and batteries

Clinical features (depending on location):

◆ Flinching with sharp pain on swallowing
◆ Drooling saliva
◆ Airway compromise/cough
◆ Voice change
◆ Neck emphysema/mediastinitis if perforated

Diagnosis and localisation of foreign bodies

◆ Detailed history and description of symptoms – pain above the cricoid is an accurate indicator of the object's location, and the object should be visible on nasoendoscopy. Pain behind the sternum may indicate oesophageal location.
◆ Examination of neck and oropharynx – looking for emphysema.
◆ Lateral neck X-ray – this may prove helpful for radio-opaque foreign bodies but often leads to confusion in the case of fish bones. Increased prevertebral shadow or air in the oesophagus may point to the presence of a foreign body.
◆ Flexible nasoendoscopy – this can survey the area down to vocal folds/hypopharynx.
◆ Barium swallow – this may help in the case of a radiolucent body.
◆ Failure to locate the foreign body should not be a deterrent to initiating treatment in the case of clear history, signs or symptoms.

Treatment by location

◆ Oropharyngeal – the foreign body may be removed using a local anaesthetic spray and McGill's forceps, with or without the aid of an intubating laryngoscope.
◆ Hypopharyngeal – local anaesthetic spray and forceps may be used to remove the foreign body, but direct pharyngoscopy under anaesthetic may be necessary.
◆ Oesophageal – soft boluses may be treated initially with hyoscine butylbromide (Buscopan®) in the hope that muscle relaxation may lead to passage of the bolus. However direct oesophagoscopy under anaesthetic may be required if there is no progress, and this should be done early to reduce the risk of perforation. Foreign bodies usually settle at one of the three natural stenoses of the oesophagus: cricopharyngeus muscle; external impingement of aortic arch and left main bronchus; and cardia of the stomach. Pathological stenoses may also be present.
◆ Laryngeal/tracheal – a rigid or flexible bronchoscopy may be necessary to remove the foreign body; those that cannot be removed by this method may require referral to a cardiothoracic team for further management and thoracotomy.
◆ Patients with repeated foreign body lodgement will require a barium swallow assessment.

Direct laryngo/pharyngo/oesophagoscopy

A pharyngoscope or oesophagoscope is inserted under anaesthetic to survey the larynx and pharynx, including the vocal cords. The cricopharyngeal sphincter is then visualised and gently entered, and the oesophagus slowly followed down until the foreign body is located. It may be pushed further downwards or retrieved. Postoperatively the patient should be assessed for perforation before oral intake is permitted. Tachycardia and pyrexia may be early signs of perforation, indicating the need for radio-opaque swallow and possible repair.

6   Paediatric Otolaryngology

PAEDIATRIC ANATOMY

Paediatric ENT anatomy differs from adults in a number of respects.

Waldeyer's ring

Waldeyer's ring of lymphoepithelial tissue consists of:

◆ pharyngeal tonsils (adenoids)
◆ tubal tonsil (around eustachian tube cushion)
◆ palatine tonsil
◆ lingual tonsil (at the base of the tongue).

Development of Waldeyer's ring of lymphoepithelial tissue in the pharynx happens rapidly between the first and third years of a child's life, and makes the palatine, lingual and tubal tonsils and the adenoids relatively large compared with the lumen of the naso- and oropharynx. This may commonly lead to obstructive or infective problems in the pharynx, which may be best solved by removal. This lymphoepithelial tissue peaks in size around the seventh year and then begins to atrophy, although problems may continue well into teenage years. However, the changing nature of the tissue means that in children it is often wise to 'wait and watch' for a few months before committing a child to an operation.

Eustachian tube

The eustachian tube in children is short, straight and wide, leaving it more prone to infection and hence otitis media. It is also more likely to be dysfunctional in children, leading to inadequate equalisation and consequent otitis media with effusion (glue ear), which has a peak incidence between 3 and 6 years of age. Glue ear has a typical picture of a grey or yellow membrane, with a fluid level visible on occasions. A flat type-B tympanogram accompanied by conductive hearing loss is typical, and parents or school staff may report an apparent hearing loss.

Larynx

The larynx of a neonate is relatively floppy, and this may lead to stridor at, or immediately after, birth. This is due to the in-drawing of aryepiglottic folds on inspiration, and in some cases it may be helpful to perform an aryepiglottoplasty in order to remove any lax tissue. In most cases, however, conservative management results in eventual resolution over a number of months or years.

PAEDIATRIC ENT CONDITIONS

Acute epiglottitis

- A bacterial infection of the throat characterised by progressive acute laryngitis which affects all the supraglottis, but predominately the loose connective tissue of the epiglottis.
- Usually caused by *H. influenzae* type B, but staphylococci, β-haemolytic streptococci and pneumococci have all been found.

Clinical features

- Usually occurs in children aged 2–7 years.
- Initially the child complains of a sore throat which rapidly progresses to inspiratory stridor.
- Pyrexia (temperature of 38–40 °C).
- The child tends to lean forwards and drools.

Do not attempt to examine the child as this may precipitate laryngospasm

Management

- The child's airway must be secured.
- An experienced paediatric anaesthetist and otolaryngologist must be in·attendance.
- Child and parent are moved to an induction area with operating facilities adjacent.
- Anaesthesia is induced by inhalation.
- An endotracheal tube is passed; at this time, a cherry-red epiglottis will be seen.
- Rigid bronchoscopy can be used to intubate if initial attempts at intubation fail.
- Tracheostomy is rarely required.
- Intravenous access, blood cultures and throat swabs are performed after the airway has been secured.
- Patients respond quickly to iv antibiotics (eg chloramphenicol) and usually can be extubated after 24–48 hours.
- Steroids may be of value before decannulation to reduce oedema.

The incidence of acute epiglottitis in children has been declining, which may be due to HiB vaccination.

Congenital hearing problems

Syndromic hearing loss

Many syndromes are associated with a sensorineural, conductive or mixed hearing loss:

- Pendred's syndrome – autosomal recessive syndrome involving sensorineural hearing loss with thyroid goitre.
- Treacher Collins' syndrome – autosomal dominant (AD) syndrome with characteristic underdevelopment of maxilla and mandible, along with microtia and other ear abnormalities.
- Pierre Robin syndrome – AD syndrome involving hypoplastic mandible with cleft palate and ear deformities.
- Crouzon's disease – AD syndrome, hypoplastic mandible and maxilla, craniostenosis, exophthalmos and ear abnormalities.
- Apert's syndrome – AD syndrome, syndactyly, cleft palate, maxillary underdevelopment, stapes footplate fixation.

Dysplasias

Congenital dysplasias such as Mondini's dysplasia affect the development of the cochlea, leading to sensorineural deafness.

Intrauterine disease

Hearing may be lost due to disease in the womb, for example due to rubella, or perinatal disorders (such as hypoxia or prematurity).

Congenital disorders predisposing to glue ear

Down's syndrome, cleft palate and cystic fibrosis increase the risk of glue ear.

Airway problems

A number of conditions, including trauma and inhaled foreign bodies may cause airway problems in children. The following are also important causes of airway difficulties in children:

- **Laryngomalacia** – this commonly manifests soon after birth, and represents the indrawing of the underdeveloped larynx as mentioned above. An aryepiglottoplasty may be required. However, most cases settle without intervention.
- **Vocal cord paralysis** – this usually has to be bilateral to cause symptoms. There is an abductor paralysis and stridor is common, with no effect on the voice. Most recover in a few years, but a few require tracheostomy or surgical treatment of the paralysis.
- **Laryngotracheobronchitis** – infection causes inspiratory stridor and oedema, and in the worst cases intubation is necessary. Treatment is with antibiotics, and extubation follows.

- **Subglottic stenosis** – the subglottis may be narrowed by scar tissue after intubation, and a cricoid split may be necessary, with or without insertion of a cartilage graft to widen the lumen.
- **Laryngeal papillomatosis** – there are extensive papillomas around the larynx. Immunity develops with age but, in the meantime, laser treatment may be necessary.
- **Subglottic haemangioma** – this and other space-occupying lesions may affect the paediatric airway and may need surgical or laser removal.
- **Laryngeal web** – this may be congenital or acquired. It may be managed conservatively or treated surgically.
- **Choanal atresia** – failure of breakdown of the bucconasal membrane in utero blocks the airway, and if bilateral leads to breathing difficulty at birth as neonates are obligate nasal breathers. Choanal atresia may be associated with other abnormalities (the CHARGE association – **C**oloboma, **H**eart disease, **A**tresia, **R**etarded growth, **G**enital abnormalities and **E**ar abnormalities). Surgery may be required to perforate the occlusion, and repeat dilation and treatment may be required to keep the lumen patent in the early years.

Adenoids

- Also known as pharyngeal tonsils.
- Mass of lymphoid tissue at postero-superior nasopharynx.
- Maximum relative size between the ages of 3 and 8 years.
- Thought to play a role in 'sampling' of ingested/inhaled substances and production of antibodies.
- Inflammation may be due to acute infections.
- May cause nasal obstruction, snoring, sleep apnoea and hyponasal speech.
- May cause eustachian tube dysfunction and glue ear.

Investigations

- Audiometry/tympanogram
- Lateral soft tissue neck X-ray
- Postnasal space mirror
- Fibreoptic nasoendoscope examination
- Examination under anaesthetic

Indications for adenoidectomy

- Nasal obstruction
- Glue ear
- Recurrent acute otitis media
- Rhinosinusitis
- Sleep apnoea

Contraindications for adenoidectomy

◆ Recent upper respiratory tract infection
◆ Bleeding disorder
◆ Cleft palate/submucous cleft (may lead to nasal regurgitation)

Procedure

After insertion of a Boyle–Davis gag the adenoids are assessed, and a curette, or a suction diathermy catheter with a mirror, is used to remove them. Haemostasis is achieved with suction diathermy, packing and adrenaline swabs.

Complications

◆ Bleeding – generally from the ascending pharyngeal or sphenopalatine arteries, treated in the same way as a post-tonsillectomy haemorrhage
◆ Hypernasal speech
◆ Nasal regurgitation
◆ Regrowth of adenoid tissue
◆ Damage to soft palate/teeth

PAEDIATRIC HEARING TESTS AND SCREENING

At present all children are screened for hearing at the following ages:

◆ 7 months – distraction testing
◆ 2–4 years – distraction tests or conditioned responses
◆ > 5 years – pure tone audiometry

The full range of subjective and objective hearing tests includes the following:

◆ Otoacoustic emissions (OAEs) – measurement of distortion product OAEs is being developed as a universal hearing screening tool for very young children.
◆ Auditory response cradle – this monitors head turning, startle responses, body movements and respiratory changes in response to sound stimuli.
◆ Distraction testing – the child's responses are noted to sounds made out of view on either side, while the child is distracted by play.
◆ Conditioned response audiometry – the child is 'trained' to perform a task after hearing a particular auditory stimulus. The stimulus is then applied from various directions and at varying volumes.
◆ Speech discrimination testing – the child is asked to point to a number of objects, with names designed to sound very similar.
◆ Pure tone audiometry – this can be performed on children 4 years of age and older in a manner similar to adults.

SECTION

2

Practice Questions

CONTENTS

EMQs

CONTENTS

The following pages provide practice Extended Matching Questions, with answers and brief explanations given later. The questions cover some areas not included in the revision text and, as such, are an additional revision resource.

You should read all answer options carefully before considering each stem in turn. Remember that answer options may be used more than once. For further revision, you may find it helpful to devise your own EMQs.

Extended Matching Questions (EMQs)

1 BASIC SCIENCES

1.1 Peripheral nerve anatomy

A Facial nerve	**E** Cranial accessory nerve
B Lingual nerve	**F** Oculomotor nerve
C Ophthalmic nerve	**G** Glossopharyngeal nerve
D Trochlear nerve	**H** Cervical sympathetic trunk

For each of the patients below, select the nerve most likely to be involved from the list above. Each option may be used once, more than once or not at all.

☐ **1** Two days after a left lower wisdom tooth extraction, a fit 23-year-old man complains of a severe bleed from the left side of his tongue, which he has bitten. The tongue is insensitive to touch and taste stimuli on the left.

☐ **2** A fit 26-year-old man suddenly develops a persistent dry left eye, clouded vision, blunted taste sensation and an inability to empty food from the left vestibule.

☐ **3** A 40-year-old woman complains of clouded vision in her left eye after development of a rash over the left side of her forehead. She has burning pain over her left forehead and in her left eye, but no ptosis or diplopia. The corneal reflex is intact.

1.2 Selection of drains for surgical procedures

A Sump
B Corrugated
C Suction
D Tube drain
E None

For each of the operations listed below, select the single most appropriate drain from the list above. Each answer may be used once, more than once, or not at all.

☐ **1** Thyroidectomy.

☐ **2** Drainage of a large pinna haematoma.

☐ **3** Radical neck dissection.

☐ **4** Myringoplasty.

1.3 Nutrition

A Nasogastric feeding
B Jejunostomy feeding
C Parenteral nutrition
D Omega fatty acid feed
E Elemental diet

Select the most appropriate nutritional approach for each of the patients below. Each option may be used once, more than once, or not at all.

☐ **1** A 34-year-old woman suffers an acute attack of absolute dysphagia, which is diagnosed as being due to severe tonsillitis. She begins to recover with iv antibiotics.

☐ **2** A 76-year-old man had a total pharyngolaryngo-oesophagectomy for squamous cell carcinoma. The procedure is expected to be curative, but the patient lost 20% of his weight in the 3 months before the operation.

1.4 Consent for surgical treatment

A Yes, surgery can proceed
B No, surgery cannot proceed
C Apply to make the child a ward of court
D Obtain consent from his wife
E Obtain consent from the patient

For each of the situations below, select the most likely answer from the list above. Each option may be used once, more than once, or not at all.

☐ **1** A 74-year-old man found unconscious at home is brought in by ambulance. It is evident that his consciousness level has deteriorated because of a brisk uncontrolled epistaxis, and he is unable to give consent to an examination under anaesthetic and a ligation of the sphenopalatine artery. His wife has been contacted and is at the hospital, but has expressed her refusal to allow him to be operated on. Would you proceed against her wishes?

☐ **2** A member of a religious sect has brought in his 11-year-old son with bleeding post-tonsillectomy. The bleeding is not controlled with conservative measures, and he needs to go to theatre for arrest of bleeding, but both parents adamantly refuse, saying that he will get better through the fervent prayers of members of his sect. Despite attempts at persuasion, they refuse to give consent for surgery. What option is available to the surgeon?

☐ **3** A 35-year-old woman with a severe psychiatric illness swallows a chicken bone, which lodges in her oesophagus and prevents her from eating and drinking. Her psychiatrist agrees with the ENT opinion that she requires urgent removal of the bone under anaesthetic. Her psychiatric state does not allow her to give informed consent for the procedure. What process should follow?

☐ **4** A 70-year-old man with a maxillary sinus tumour and cerebral metastases refuses any surgery and expresses his wish formally in writing. He is judged to be mentally competent. The following day he enters into a coma and his wife, who was abroad, arrives at his bedside and demands that surgical treatment is commenced. Can surgery proceed?

1.5 Micro-organisms

A *Escherichia coli*
B *Streptococcus pneumoniae*
C *Clostridium difficile*
D *Staphylococcus aureus*

E *Haemophilus influenzae*
F *Clostridium perfringens*
G None of the above

From the list above, choose the most common causative organism for the following infections. Each may be used once, more than once, or not at all.

☐ **1** Ludwig's angina.

☐ **2** Vincent's angina.

☐ **3** Postoperative diarrhoea.

1.6 Anticoagulant treatment regimens

A Warfarin to maintain an INR of 2–3
B Unfractionated heparin 5000 IU subcutaneously bd
C Unfractionated heparin iv to maintain an APTT ratio of 2.5–3.5
D Tinzaparin 3500 U once daily
E Tinzaparin 175 U/kg once daily

For each of the clinical scenarios below, select the most appropriate anticoagulation regimen to initiate treatment from the options listed above. Each option may be used once, more than once or not at all.

☐ **1** A 34-year-old woman with factor V Leiden but no previous history of venous thrombosis is admitted for nasal polypectomy. A previous polypectomy was complicated by excessive bleeding.

☐ **2** A 76-year-old man develops a popliteal vein thrombosis 5 days after a total laryngectomy.

☐ **3** A 45-year-old man takes warfarin because he has a prosthetic heart valve, and attends the ward 3 days before an elective total thyroidectomy.

1.7 Treatment of bleeding in an anticoagulated patient

A Cessation of anticoagulation therapy and observation
B Vitamin K im
C Fresh frozen plasma 30 ml/kg alone
D Vitamin K iv and fresh frozen plasma 30 ml/kg
E Vitamin K alone iv
F Protamine sulphate iv
G Oral protamine sulphate and observation

For each of the clinical scenarios below, select the appropriate measure to correct the haemostatic abnormality from the list above. Each option may be used once, more than once or not at all.

☐ **1** A 56-year-old man, who has been taking warfarin for atrial fibrillation for 4 years, recently received a course of oral antibiotics from his GP for a chest infection. His INR is 8.0. He now presents with life-threatening epistaxis.

☐ **2** A 28-year-old woman with a prosthetic mitral valve has recently undergone an elective thyroidectomy. Preoperatively, her warfarin was discontinued and she was established on an iv heparin infusion. Immediately before theatre, her INR was 1.3 and her APTT ratio was 2.0. At 12 hours postoperatively, she develops severe bleeding from her wound. Her INR is now 1.1 and her APTT ratio 6.0.

1.8 Suture materials

A Absorbable, braided, synthetic
B Absorbable, monofilament, synthetic
C Non-absorbable, braided, natural material
D Non-absorbable, monofilament, synthetic

For each of the suture materials listed below, select the most appropriate description from the list above. Each option may be used once, more than once, or not at all.

☐ **1** Polyglactic acid (Vicryl®).

☐ **2** Nylon.

☐ **3** Polyglyconate (Maxon®).

☐ **4** Polypropylene (Prolene®).

☐ **5** Polydioxanone (PDS®).

☐ **6** Polyglycolic acid (Dexon®).

☐ **7** Silk.

2 AUDIOLOGY

2.1 Conditions

A Ménière's disease
B Glue ear
C Presbyacusis
D Noise-induced hearing loss

E Acoustic neuroma
F Perforation
G Congenital hearing loss

Which of the above conditions is being described here? Each option may be used once, more than once or not at all.

☐ 1 A 45-year-old man suffers episodic vertigo and tinnitus, with gradually decreasing hearing.

☐ 2 A 60-year-old man has bilateral hearing loss at a frequency of around 4–6 Hz.

☐ 3 A 60-year-old woman shows gradual progressive unilateral deafness with constant tinnitus but no vertigo.

2.2 Audiological/vestibular tests – 1

A Centrally evoked response audiometry
B Electrocochleogram
C Pure tone audiometry
D Brainstem electrical response audiometry

E Caloric testing
F Rotation testing
G Tympanometry

Which of the above audiological/vestibular tests is most appropriate in each of the following cases? Each option may be used once, more than once or not at all.

☐ 1 Assessment of a 2-year-old child to determine if glue ear is present.

☐ 2 Assessment of a 55-year-old man suspected of having a unilateral vestibular nerve lesion.

☐ 3 Intraoperative monitoring for surgery in a 75-year-old woman to remove acoustic neuroma.

2.3 Audiological/vestibular tests – 2

A Luescher's test	**E** Rinne's test
B Fowler's test	**F** Stenger's test
C Romberg's test	**G** Bing test
D Weber's test	**H** Unterberger's test

Which of the above audiological/vestibular tests is being described below? Each option may be used once, more than once or not at all.

☐ **1** A test using two tuning forks, presented to each ear simultaneously, which helps to differentiate a real from a false hearing loss.

☐ **2** A patient is asked to walk on the spot for 30 seconds with eyes closed and arms outstretched – a body rotation of greater than 30° or a movement of > 1 m is abnormal.

☐ **3** A central tuning fork heard on one side indicates a possible conductive hearing loss in that ear.

☐ **4** A tuning fork is struck and held on the mastoid process, and the patient is asked to occlude the opposite ear – if the sound becomes quieter, a conductive hearing loss is indicated.

2.4 Diagnoses

A Right-sided conductive deafness	**E** Bilateral sensorineural hearing loss
B Left-sided conductive deafness	**F** Bilateral conductive hearing loss
C Right-sided sensorineural hearing loss	**G** Normal hearing
D Left-sided sensorineural hearing loss	

Which condition from the list above is being diagnosed by the test described below? Each option may be used once, more than once or not at all.

☐ **1** Weber's test localises to the left side, and Rinne's test is negative on the left and positive on the right.

☐ **2** Weber's test localises to the right side and Rinne's test is positive on both sides.

☐ **3** Weber's test localises to the centre and Rinne's test is positive on both sides.

2.5 Audiological aids

A Cochlear implant
B Bone-anchored hearing aid
C Behind-the-ear hearing aid
D Lip-reading

E Tinnitus masker
F Cooksey–Cawthorne exercises
G Epley manoeuvre

Which of the above audiological aids would be most appropriate in the following patients? Each option may be used once, more than once or not at all.

☐ **1** A child with microtia and bilateral conductive hearing loss.

☐ **2** A 35-year-old man suffers sudden-onset violent dizziness, alternating with tinnitus and vertigo. His symptoms gradually subside but a degree of vertigo remains.

☐ **3** A 45-year-old lady suffers with a feeling of the room spinning on turning her head in a particular direction and on lying down in bed.

2.6 Audiovestibular structures

A Cochlear nerve
B Superior vestibular nerve
C Inferior vestibular nerve
D Medial geniculate body

E Cerebral cortex
F Cerebellum
G Outer hair cell mechanism
H Inner hair cell mechanism

Which of the above audiovestibular structures is being described below? Each option may be used once, more than once or not at all.

☐ **1** Supplies the lateral semicircular canals.

☐ **2** Thought to act to fine-tune hearing at a specific frequency.

☐ **3** The site of the second neural synapse in the auditory pathway.

☐ **4** Pierces the temporal bone in its anterior-inferior quadrant.

2.7 Vertigo

A Application of cold water to right ear	**E** Cerebellar lesion
B Application of cold water to left ear	**F** Labyrinthitis
C Cerebrovascular ischaemia	**G** Benign paroxysmal positional vertigo
D Ménière's disease	**H** Iatrogenic vertigo

Which of the above causes of vertigo is most likely in the cases described below? Each option may be used once, more than once or not at all.

☐ **1** A 35-year-old man experiences a 3-day period of constant vertigo accompanied by nausea and vomiting. This settles with symptomatic treatment. Dix–Hallpike testing provokes no return of symptoms.

☐ **2** A 55-year-old woman suffers intermittent episodes of vertigo, exacerbated by lying down.

☐ **3** A 65-year-old man suffers an episode of acute vertigo lasting for 12 hours, and this is accompanied by a left-sided weakness that resolves.

☐ **4** A 40-year-old woman experiences intermittent vertigo lasting about half an hour each time, and accompanied by some nausea. Over the last few years she has noticed a deterioration in her hearing.

☐ **5** During a medical procedure, a patient experiences temporary nystagmus to the left.

3 OTOLOGY

3.1 Anatomy

A Greater auricular nerve	**E** Posterior auricular nerve
B Alderman's/Arnold's nerve	**F** Tympanic nerve
C Jacobson's nerve	**G** Chorda tympani
D Auriculotemporal nerve	

Which of the above nerves supplies the following areas? Each option may be used once, more than once or not at all.

☐ **1** The upper lateral surface of the pinna.

☐ **2** The sensory supply to the middle ear.

☐ **3** May be stimulated in the external auditory meatus to cause coughing.

3.2 Micro-organisms

A Streptococcus pneumoniae	E Staphylococcus albans
B Haemophilus influenzae	F Epstein–Barr virus
C Staphylococcus aureus	G Respiratory syncytial virus
D Pseudomonas spp.	H Moraxella catarrhalis

Which of the above organisms is most likely to be present in the following scenarios? Each option may be used once, more than once or not at all.

☐ **1** Sudden onset of a painful ear with deafness.

☐ **2** A constant deep otalgia with evidence of cranial nerve involvement in a diabetic patient.

☐ **3** A tonsillitis lasting 2 weeks, associated with an enlarged liver.

3.3 Antibiotics

A Augmentin	E Erythromycin
B Penicillin	F Metronidazole
C Flucloxacillin	G Gentamicin
D Ciprofloxacin	

Which of the above antibiotics is most suitable as a first-line treatment in the following patients? Each option may be used once, more than once or not at all.

☐ **1** A patient with swollen tonsils and difficulty swallowing.

☐ **2** A patient with an external ear infection.

☐ **3** A patient with a painful ear, reduced hearing and some asymmetry of his pinna.

3.4 Chronic suppurative otitis media

A Lateral sinus thrombosis	**F** Tympanosclerosis
B Intracranial abscess	**G** Gradenigo's syndrome
C Meningitis	**H** Labyrinthitis
D Extradural abscess	**I** Facial nerve palsy
E Otitic hydrocephalus	

Which of the above complications of chronic suppurative otitis media is the most likely to explain the following histories? Each option may be used once, more than once or not at all.

☐ **1** A patient with an acute ear infection develops pain in the distribution of the trigeminal nerve, and some asymmetry of eye movement.

☐ **2** A patient with multiple ear infections gradually develops a moderate hearing loss.

☐ **3** A patient with sudden-onset dizziness and nausea, with nystagmus towards the affected side.

3.5 Embryology

A First pharyngeal arch	**E** Third pharyngeal arch
B First pharyngeal pouch	**F** Fourth pharyngeal arch
C Second pharyngeal arch	**G** Sixth pharyngeal arch
D Second pharyngeal pouch	

Which is the embryological origin of each of the following structures? Each option may be used once, more than once or not at all.

☐ **1** Mandible.

☐ **2** Stapes.

☐ **3** Pinna.

☐ **4** Superior parathyroid glands.

3.6 Temporal bone

A Squamous temporal bone
B Petrous temporal bone
C Stylomastoid foramen
D Tympanic plate of temporal bone
E Zygomatic temporal bone

Which of the above constituents of the temporal bone contains each of the following structures? Each option may be used once, more than once or not at all.

☐ **1** The exit point of the facial nerve.

☐ **2** The temporomandibular joint.

☐ **3** The cartilaginous eustachian tube.

☐ **4** The bony external auditory meatus.

3.7 Pathology

A Tullio phenomenon   **D** Hitselberger sign
B Fistula sign   **E** Schwartze's sign
C Gradenigo's syndrome   **F** Ramsay Hunt syndrome

Which of the above otological pathologies best fits each description below? Each option may be used once, more than once or not at all.

☐ **1** A 40-year-old lady suffers with intermittent vertigo in the presence of loud sounds.

☐ **2** A 75-year-old lady with a unilateral hearing loss and a hypoaesthesia of the ear canal on the same side.

☐ **3** A 35-year-old lady suffers with deafness, tinnitus and vertigo; on examination there is a pink tinge to the tympanic membrane.

3.8 Middle ear nerves

A Facial nerve	**E** Lesser petrosal nerve
B Tympanic nerve	**F** Caroticotympanic nerve
C Tympanic plexus	**G** Auricular branch of the vagus nerve
D Chorda tympani	

Which of the above middle ear nerves is being described below? Each option may be used once, more than once or not at all.

☐ **1** Arises from the glossopharyngeal nerve just below the jugular foramen. It grooves the surface of the promontory and then splits into branches.

☐ **2** Contains secretomotor fibres to the parotid gland. It passes through a small opening on the anterior petrous temporal bone and leaves the skull through the foramen ovale to join the otic ganglion.

☐ **3** Arises from the facial nerve above the stylomastoid foramen. It enters the tympanic cavity at the posterior border of the tympanic membrane and runs forward, around the root of the malleus handle. It leaves the tympanic cavity through the petro-tympanic fissure to enter the infratemporal fossa.

3.9 Diagnoses

A Acoustic neuroma	**F** Chronic serous otitis media
B Acute middle ear effusion	**G** Foreign body in the ear
C Acute suppurative otitis media	**H** Otitis externa
D Barotraumatic otitis media	**I** Otosclerosis
E Cholesteatoma	**J** Wax

For the patients below, select the most appropriate diagnosis from the above list. Each option may be used once, more than once or not at all.

☐ **1** A 32-year-old man presents with deafness and discomfort in his left ear on return from a recent summer holiday where he swam in the hotel swimming pool.

☐ **2** A 26-year-old man presents with a short history of pain made worse by jaw movements, and discharge from the ear. There is pus in the external ear canal and the skin of the canal is erythematous, swollen and tender.

☐ **3** A 60-year-old man presents with deafness and a feeling of pressure in the left ear. There is retraction of the tympanic membrane with Rinne's test negative on the left and Weber's test lateralising to the left. Posterior rhinoscopy reveals a large exophytic tumour.

☐ **4** A 45-year-old man has a 1-year-history of foul-smelling purulent discharge from the left ear and increasing deafness. There is an attic perforation, which is occupied by a greyish substance.

☐ **5** A 20-year-old woman has a 1-year history of bilateral deafness and tinnitus. The deafness is worse on the right and less marked when there is background noise. The patient's father has worn a hearing aid since his late teens.

☐ **6** A 45-year-old woman has a left-sided deafness of 5 years' duration. There is an absent left corneal reflex and some ataxia.

4 RHINOLOGY

4.1 Anatomy

A Ethmoidal bone	**E** Sphenoid bone
B Nasal bone	**F** Vomer
C Frontal process of maxilla	**G** Palatine bone
D Lacrimal bone	**H** Frontal bone

Which of the above bones is being described in the following statements? Each option may be used once, more than once or not at all.

☐ **1** Makes up the majority of the middle turbinate.

☐ **2** Makes up the inferior bony septum.

☐ **3** Is breached to get access to the frontal sinus.

4.2 Epistaxis

A Traumatic	**E** Leukaemia
B Hereditary haemorrhagic telangiectasia	**F** Haemophilia
C Drug-related	**G** Liver failure
D Angiofibroma	

Which of the above is the most likely to be the cause of epistaxis in the following cases? Each option may be used once, more than once or not at all.

☐ **1** A patient with red spots on her lips suffers from regular nosebleeds – she is also under treatment for gut lesions.

☐ **2** A male teenager suffers with repeated torrential nosebleeds, leading to anaemia. There is also chronic nasal obstruction by a hard mass.

☐ **3** A 75-year-old former alcoholic suffers continual nosebleeds – on clotting screen he is found to have a raised INR despite being on no medication.

4.3 Arteries

A Transverse cervical artery	**E** Ascending pharyngeal artery
B Sphenopalatine artery	**F** Superficial temporal artery
C Superior labial artery	**G** Lingual artery
D Anterior ethmoidal artery	**H** Superior thyroid artery

Which artery is being described in the following case scenarios? Each option may be used once, more than once or not at all.

☐ **1** A patient with intractable epistaxis has an endoscopic operation carried out where this artery is clipped off.

☐ **2** A patient with severe posterior epistaxis has this artery clipped off via a medial orbital incision.

☐ **3** A patient has acute anterior inferior epistaxis that responds quickly to pressure.

4.4 Imaging techniques

A CT scan	**E** Nucleotide scanning
B MRI scan	**F** Positron emission tomography (PET) scan
C Ultrasound scan	**G** Barium swallow
D Plain X-ray	

Which of the imaging techniques is most appropriate as a first-line scan for the following conditions? Each option may be used once, more than once or not at all.

☐ **1** Sinusitis.

☐ **2** Orbital cellulitis.

☐ **3** Suspected pharyngeal pouch.

☐ **4** Laryngeal nerve palsy.

4.5 Diagnoses

A Antrochoanal polyp	**D** Rhinitis medicamentosa
B Allergic rhinitis	**E** Rhinosinusitis
C Intrinsic rhinitis	**F** Nasal trauma

Which of the above diagnoses best fits the description below? Each option may be used once, more than once or not at all.

☐ **1** A 40-year-old man suffers with nasal obstruction and rhinorrhoea and multiple polyps. However there is no hypersensitivity to any identifiable substance.

☐ **2** A 50-year-old woman has had a long history of nasal problems, and has had long-term medical treatment for this. Over the last few months she has found bilateral congestion getting worse, despite medication.

☐ **3** A 25-year-old man with gradual-onset unilateral nasal obstruction, worse on expiration, with some ipsilateral hearing loss.

4.6 Interventions

A Septoplasty	**E** Bilateral antral washout
B Septorhinoplasty	**F** Conservative medical treatment
C Submucosal diathermy	**G** Vidian neurectomy
D Polypectomy	

Which of the above interventions is indicated in the following cases? Each option may be used once, more than once or not at all.

☐ **1** A 25-year-old male rugby player has long-standing nasal deviation to the left, nasal obstruction and breathing difficulties. A nasal manipulation has been attempted previously without success.

☐ **2** A 40-year-old woman presents with a 3-month history of chronic head pain and nasal obstruction, for which she has had no treatment.

☐ **3** A 50-year-old asthmatic man presents with a 2-year history of increasing head pain, pressure and a postnasal drip.

4.7 Taste sensation

A Filiform papillae	**D** Trigeminal nerve
B Vallate papillae	**E** Foliate papillae
C Olfactory epithelium	**F** Fungiform papillae

Which of the above structures detects the sensation described below? Each option may be used once, more than once, or not at all.

☐ **1** Sour taste.

☐ **2** Salty taste.

☐ **3** Pepper taste.

4.8 Relations

A Bulla ethmoidalis	**F** Maxillary sinus
B Ethmoid sinus	**G** Middle concha
C Eustachian tube	**H** Sphenoid sinus
D Frontal sinus	**I** Superior concha
E Inferior concha	**J** Vestibule

Which of the above has the following relations? Each option may be used once, more than once or not at all.

☐ **1** A posterior relation to the supraciliary arch.

☐ **2** Is related inferiorly to the molar teeth.

☐ **3** Is a medial relation to the orbit.

☐ **4** Is an inferior relation to the pituitary gland.

☐ **5** Is a medial relation of the nasolacrimal duct.

4.9 Diagnoses

A Allergic rhinitis	**F** Osler–Weber–Rendu disease
B Drug-induced	**G** Pyogenic granuloma
C Foreign body	**H** Thrombocytopenic purpura
D Leukaemia	**I** Trauma
E Malignant neoplasm	**J** Wegener's granuloma

Please select the most appropriate diagnosis for the patients below from the above list. Each option may be used once, more than once or not at all.

☐ **1** A 3-year-old has bleeding from one side of the nose, along with a foul-smelling discharge.

☐ **2** A 21-year-old man has unilateral epistaxis. He has had a history of malaise and breathlessness for some weeks, and is clinically anaemic despite only losing a small amount of blood.

☐ **3** An elderly man has epistaxis. He recently had open-heart surgery with placement of a prosthetic mitral valve.

☐ **4** A young woman presents with epistaxis. Anterior rhinoscopy reveals a smooth swollen red mass with contact bleeding.

☐ **5** A middle-aged man has a long history of repeated heavy epistaxes. The mucous membrane of his nose has several red spots on both sides. Inspection of his nose and face reveals similar spots that are dilated capillaries.

5 LARYNGOLOGY

5.1 Nerve damage

A Recurrent laryngeal nerve
B External branch of the superior laryngeal nerve
C Internal branch of the superior laryngeal nerve
D Phrenic nerve
E Vagus nerve
F Accessory nerve
G Glossopharyngeal nerve
H Hypoglossal nerve
I Lingual nerve

Which of the above nerves is most likely to have been damaged in the following cases? Each option may be used once, more than once or not at all.

☐ **1** After a radical neck dissection, a patient finds difficulty in shrugging his shoulders.

☐ **2** After thyroid surgery, a patient develops a weak, hoarse voice.

☐ **3** After submandibular gland excision, a patient develops deviation of the tongue on protrusion.

5.2 Foramina

A Optic canal
B Superior orbital fissure
C Foramen rotundum
D Foramen ovale
E Foramen spinosum

F Foramen lacerum
G Jugular foramen
H Hypoglossal canal
I Foramen magnum

Which of the above foramina transmits the following structures? Each option may be used once, more than once or not at all.

☐ **1** The maxillary nerve.

☐ **2** The glossopharyngeal nerve.

☐ **3** The spinal root of the accessory nerve, but not the cervical root.

5.3 Muscles

A Palatoglossus	**F** Omohyoid
B Palatopharyngeus	**G** Sternohyoid
C Styloglossus	**H** Palatoglossus
D Tensor veli palati	**I** Hyoglossus
E Levator veli palati	

Which of the above muscles is being described in the following statements? Each option may be used once, more than once or not at all.

☐ **1** This muscle is supplied by the mandibular branch of the trigeminal nerve, and attaches to the medial pterygoid plate and to the auditory tube cartilage, running to the palate.

☐ **2** This internal pharyngeal muscle is supplied by the vagus nerve and runs between the superior and middle constrictors.

☐ **3** This is an extrinsic muscle of the tongue.

5.4 Histological diagnoses

A Adenocarcinoma	**E** Chemodectoma
B Squamous cell carcinoma	**F** Adenolymphoma
C Mucoepidermoid carcinoma	**G** Pleomorphic adenoma
D Adenoid cystic carcinoma	

Which of the above histological diagnoses is most likely in the following cases? Each option may be used once, more than once or not at all.

☐ **1** A retired mahogany worker develops epistaxis, nasal obstruction and proptosis.

☐ **2** A middle-aged man develops a hard swelling below his ear with some paralysis of his mouth.

☐ **3** A 40-year-old woman develops a firm swelling below her ear, but without any facial asymmetry.

5.5 Facial nerve palsy

A Cerebrovascular accident
B Bell's palsy
C Ramsay Hunt syndrome
D Trauma

E Glomus tumour
F Parotid malignancy
G Multiple sclerosis

Which of the above causes is most likely in each of the following cases of facial nerve palsy? Each option may be used once, more than once or not at all.

☐ **1** A 50-year-old man develops facial asymmetry in association with severe ear pain and dizziness, with some vesicles visible in the ear.

☐ **2** A 64-year-old woman develops intermittent facial palsy, as well as intermittent blindness and weakness. The disease is slowly progressive.

☐ **3** A 40-year-old woman develops a facial asymmetry that affects her forehead 2 weeks after a severe viral infection.

5.6 Neck lumps

A Plunging ranula
B Chemodectoma
C Branchial cyst
D Thyroid lump

E Thyroglossal cyst
F Parotid neoplasm
G Dermoid cyst

Which one of the above neck lumps best fits the description below? Each option may be used once, more than once or not at all.

☐ **1** A 50-year-old Nepalese man presents with a lump in the area of the carotid artery bifurcation.

☐ **2** A 25-year-old student develops sudden onset of painless swelling underneath the sternocleidomastoid muscle.

☐ **3** A 6-year-old child is noted to have a central neck lump, which moves with swallowing and tongue protrusion.

5.7 Thyroid neoplasms

A Follicular carcinoma	**D** Medullary carcinoma
B Follicular adenoma	**E** Anaplastic carcinoma
C Papillary adenoma	**F** Lymphoma

Which one of the above thyroid neoplasms best fits the descriptions below? Each option may be used once, more than once or not at all.

☐ **1** A 34-year-old woman has previously suffered with a tumour of the adrenal medulla, and develops a neck lump.

☐ **2** A 55-year-old woman who has previously suffered from iodine deficiency develops a solitary thyroid lump.

☐ **3** An 85-year-old woman who is known to have a goitre develops a rapidly enlarging neck lump.

5.8 Surgical complications

A Superficial parotidectomy	**D** Tonsillectomy
B Radical neck dissection	**E** Stapedectomy
C Submandibular gland dissection	**F** Functional endoscopic sinus surgery

Which of the above operations is most commonly associated with the complications described below? Each option may be used once, more than once or not at all.

☐ **1** A 40-year-old man, 6 months after the operation, finds that when he chews, his cheek sweats profusely.

☐ **2** A 50-year-old man suffers a sudden deterioration in vision immediately after his operation.

☐ **3** A 67-year-old man finds it is difficult to shrug his shoulder postoperatively.

☐ **4** A 55-year-old woman finds that her face has become asymmetrical immediately postoperatively.

5.9 Thyroid cancer

A Papillary carcinoma	**D** Anaplastic carcinoma
B Follicular carcinoma	**E** Lymphoma
C Medullary cell carcinoma	**F** Thyroid secondaries from another primary organ

For each of the statements below, select the correct thyroid carcinoma from the list above. Each option may be used once, more than once or not at all.

☐ **1** Has early haematogenous and lymphatic spread.

☐ **2** Is usually very radiosensitive.

☐ **3** Accounts for 60% of thyroid carcinomas.

☐ **4** Is derived from parafollicular C cells.

☐ **5** Commonly metastasises to bone and lung, with lymphatic spread being unusual.

6 PAEDIATRICS

6.1 Airway difficulty

A Asthma	**F** Foreign body
B Adenotonsillar enlargement	**G** Central apnoea
C Choanal atresia	**H** Cystic hygroma
D Laryngomalacia	**I** Vocal cord palsy
E Subglottic stenosis	

Which of the above causes of paediatric airway difficulty is most likely in the following cases? Each option may be used once, more than once or not at all.

☐ **1** At birth, a baby boy presents with immediate difficulty in breathing, despite respiratory effort.

☐ **2** After prolonged intubation, a 4-year-old boy develops chronic stridor requiring further intubation and surgical intervention.

☐ **3** A 1-year-old infant has a tendency to stridulous breathing, which seems to be slowly improving with time.

6.2 Airway interventions

A Nasal prong	**E** Choanal atresia repair
B Laryngotracheal reconstruction	**F** Bronchodilators
C Tonsillectomy	**G** Tracheal stenting
D Tracheostomy	**H** Steroids

Which of the above airway interventions would be most helpful for the following children? Each option may be used once, more than once or not at all.

☐ **1** A child develops severe subglottic stenosis after prolonged intubation.

☐ **2** A 2-month-old infant with Pierre Robin syndrome has chronically stertorious breathing.

☐ **3** A child with obstructive sleep apnoea and grade II tonsillar hypertrophy.

6.3 Hearing tests

A Distraction testing	**E** Brainstem evoked response testing
B Pure tone audiogram	**F** Cortical evoked response testing
C Electrocochleogram	**G** Conditioned response audiometry
D Auditory response cradle	

Which of the above hearing tests is most appropriate for the children described below? Each option may be used once, more than once or not at all.

☐ **1** Testing a 6-month-old infant suspected of suffering from congenital hearing loss.

☐ **2** Screening a 7-month-old infant for hearing loss who seems to have normal hearing.

☐ **3** Assessing an unco-operative child for frequency-specific hearing thresholds.

6.4 Interventions

A Adenoidectomy
B Tonsillectomy
C Shah grommet insertion
D T-tube insertion
E No surgical intervention needed

Which of the following interventions is most appropriate in the following cases? Each option may be used once, more than once or not at all.

☐ **1** A 7-year-old boy with recurrent acute otitis media.

☐ **2** An 8-year-old girl with cleft palate, hearing loss, flat tympanograms and mild snoring.

☐ **3** A 10-year-old boy with three episodes of tonsillitis in the last year.

6.5 Diagnoses

A Epiglottitis
B Laryngotracheobronchitis
C Subglottic haemangioma
D Papillomata
E Laryngomalacia
F Anaphylaxis

Which of the above is the most likely diagnosis in the following cases? Each option can be used once, more than once or not at all.

☐ **1** A 3-year-old girl with a history of a sore throat, who now presents with a high fever and sits forward, dribbling saliva.

☐ **2** A newborn baby has an intermittent stridor from birth, but feeds and cries normally.

☐ **3** A 7-year-old boy has a varying degree of hoarseness, which is regularly treated with laser surgery.

6.6 Congenital hearing disorders

A Pendred's syndrome	**D** Apert's syndrome
B Sturge–Weber syndrome	**E** Prader–Willi syndrome
C Treacher Collins' syndrome	**F** Mondini dysplasia

Which of the above congenital hearing disorders is being described below? Each option may be used once, more than once or not at all.

☐ **1** A child with an autosomal dominant condition resulting in a cleft palate, syndactyly, fixation of the stapes footplate and maxillary hypoplasia.

☐ **2** A child with an autosomal recessive condition, sensorineural hearing loss and a thyroid goitre.

☐ **3** A child with a congenital hearing loss where the semicircular canals and most of the cochlea are absent.

6.7 Age at diagnosis

A At birth
B In the first year of life
C Between 2 and 5 years
D Between 6 and 10 years
E 10 years and above

When would the following paediatric complaints be most likely to be diagnosed? Each option may be used once, more than once or not at all.

☐ **1** Bilateral choanal atresia.

☐ **2** Subglottic stenosis.

☐ **3** Otitis media with effusion.

MTFs

CONTENTS

The following pages provide practice Multiple True/False Questions, with answers and brief explanations given later. Again, some new areas are covered with respect to the revision text and, as such, the questions are an additional revision resource.

You should read the stem carefully, and then consider each statement carefully to decide whether it is true or false. If you are not sure, it is best to guess – you will soon get a feeling for the reliability of your instincts! Devising your own MTFs may help you further.

Multiple True/False Questions (MTFs)

1 BASIC SCIENCES

1.1 Regarding anaesthetics for ENT:
☐ **A** Nitrous oxide increases middle ear pressure
☐ **B** Anaesthetic gases used in ENT surgery are flammable
☐ **C** All asthmatic patients should have a chest X-ray preoperatively
☐ **D** The laryngeal mask airway provides a secure airway

1.2 Regarding local anaesthetics:
☐ **A** They work better at low pH
☐ **B** They are a good choice for infected tissue
☐ **C** The maximum safe dose of lidocaine is 7 mg/kg
☐ **D** Prilocaine lasts longer than bupivacaine
☐ **E** Classically, Moffett's solution contains cocaine

1.3 Concerning lasers for ENT:
☐ **A** Laser light may be focused with a lens
☐ **B** NdYAG laser also provides coagulation
☐ **C** The argon laser is well absorbed by blood
☐ **D** The CO_2 laser is the most commonly used laser for throat lesions
☐ **E** All personnel must wear eye protection

1.4 Concerning medicolegal issues:
☐ **A** By attending an A&E department and asking to be seen, a patient gives a degree of implied consent
☐ **B** A doctor may decide not to mention a particular risk if he thinks it is in the patient's best interests not to do so
☐ **C** Negligence is sufficient to bring a negligence claim, whether or not damage results
☐ **D** The Bowlam test states that a practitioner avoids liability if he or she has been shown to have acted in the patient's best interests
☐ **E** Dental damage is the most common reason for ENT litigation

1.5 Regarding ENT radiology:
- ☐ **A** In MRI scanning, T2-weighted images are best for soft tissue
- ☐ **B** Lateral soft tissue X-rays are essential in the case of a suspected throat foreign body
- ☐ **C** Water-soluble contrast agents are needed if aspiration is likely
- ☐ **D** CT scanning should be used for the diagnosis of sinusitis
- ☐ **E** A chest X-ray is essential in the case of a sudden laryngeal nerve palsy

1.6 During exercise:
- ☐ **A** Cardiac output can increase sixfold
- ☐ **B** There is a decrease in PaO_2 and $PaCO_2$
- ☐ **C** Anticipation of exercise can cause an increase in respiratory rate
- ☐ **D** An increase in systolic and diastolic blood pressure is seen
- ☐ **E** Renal blood flow is increased
- ☐ **F** There is a decrease in negative intrathoracic pressure

1.7 Regarding pre-operative work-up for general anaesthetic:
- ☐ **A** All patients > 40 years of age should have an ECG
- ☐ **B** All smokers should have a chest X-ray
- ☐ **C** Premedication is not given until a consent form is signed
- ☐ **D** An FEV_1/FVC of 70% is significant

1.8 Pulse oximeters:
- ☐ **A** only sense changes in arterial blood
- ☐ **B** are unaffected by carboxyhaemoglobin
- ☐ **C** are accurate to 0.5% at > 90% oxygen saturation
- ☐ **D** may not indicate adequate ventilation
- ☐ **E** may not give accurate readings in hypovolaemic shock
- ☐ **F** are inaccurate under anaesthesia
- ☐ **G** produce false-negative results with chronic lung disease

1.9 Monopolar surgical diathermy:
- ☐ **A** utilises an alternating current of 400 Hz
- ☐ **B** requires a patient plate electrode of al least 20 cm^2
- ☐ **C** may be used for 'cutting' tissue
- ☐ **D** may be safely applied through ordinary surgical forceps
- ☐ **E** produces a local heating effect up to 1000 °C
- ☐ **F** is safer than bipolar diathermy
- ☐ **G** should not be used in patients with pacemakers
- ☐ **H** produces burn injuries that are usually partial-thickness

1.10 In a healthy adult man weighing 70 kg:
- ☐ **A** The body water content is 75%
- ☐ **B** The plasma volume is approximately 5 litres
- ☐ **C** Approximately 1.5 litres of water are lost daily from the lungs
- ☐ **D** The intracellular fluid volume is approximately two-thirds of the total body water
- ☐ **E** The daily potassium requirement is approximately 3.5–5.0 mmol/kg

1.11 Fine-needle aspiration cytology (FNAC):
☐ **A** will allow differentiation between invasive and in-situ carcinoma
☐ **B** is used to diagnose metastases
☐ **C** samples usually undergo Gram staining
☐ **D** can be used to diagnose thyroid lumps

1.12 Chronic iron deficiency anaemia:
☐ **A** produces a right shift of the oxygen dissociation curve
☐ **B** elevates the total iron-binding capacity (TIBC)
☐ **C** produces a low P_{CO_2}
☐ **D** is associated with dysphagia
☐ **E** can be associated with aspirin therapy

1.13 Regarding the coagulation cascade:
☐ **A** Synthesis of factors II, VII, IX and X is vitamin K-dependent
☐ **B** The intrinsic pathway includes factor VII
☐ **C** Fibrinogen cleaves prothrombin to yield thrombin
☐ **D** Factor VIII is synthesised mainly in the vascular endothelium
☐ **E** Antithrombin III deficiency predisposes to bleeding
☐ **F** Factor V deficiency predisposes to bleeding

1.14 In the base of the skull the:
☐ **A** foramen magnum transmits the basilar artery
☐ **B** foramen spinosum transmits cranial nerve VII
☐ **C** foramen rotundum transmits the maxillary nerve
☐ **D** foramen ovale transmits the greater petrosal nerve
☐ **E** foramen lacerum transmits the mandibular nerve

1.15 The recurrent laryngeal nerve:
☐ **A** supplies the cricothyroid muscle
☐ **B** partially supplies the trachea
☐ **C** lies alongside the inferior thyroid artery
☐ **D** should be retracted during tracheostomy to avoid damage
☐ **E** runs between the oesophagus and trachea in the neck
☐ **F** supplies the mucous surface of the vocal cords

1.16 Audit:
☐ **A** is primarily concerned with outcome analysis
☐ **B** should be led by an audit department
☐ **C** can be a process of peer review
☐ **D** only concerns doctors
☐ **E** process refers to what is done to the patient

1.17 Obtaining informed consent for a surgical procedure:

- [ ] **A** involves reference to a patient's moral rights
- [ ] **B** involves respect for patient autonomy
- [ ] **C** requires only that the patient signs a consent form after an explanation of the procedure
- [ ] **D** is unnecessary in a patient detained by Section 3 of the Mental Health Act
- [ ] **E** requires acceptance of views of children capable of expressing an opinion
- [ ] **F** involves explaining the use of invasive monitoring devices

1.18 In the setting of clinical trials:

- [ ] **A** Single-blinding refers to the patient not knowing which treatment he/she has received
- [ ] **B** Double-blinding refers to both the patient and family not knowing which treatment the patient has received
- [ ] **C** Randomisation refers to a selection process in which treatment options are decided for individual patients
- [ ] **D** Participants can withdraw even after signing a consent form
- [ ] **E** Using historical controls provides a more reliable group for comparison than a group randomised to control

2 AUDIOLOGY

2.1 With regard to acoustic neuromas:

- [ ] **A** 10% are not growing
- [ ] **B** The main otological symptom is vertigo
- [ ] **C** The most common nerve affected is the superior vestibular nerve
- [ ] **D** Hitselberger's sign is hypoaesthesia of the posterior external ear canal
- [ ] **E** They are more common in women

2.2 Regarding caloric testing:

- [ ] **A** Nystagmus is defined by the direction of the slow phase
- [ ] **B** Cold water produces nystagmus to the opposite side of infusion
- [ ] **C** Cold water is usually at 15 °C
- [ ] **D** Its effects are produced by movement of the perilymph

2.3 In the clinical assessment of hearing:

- [ ] **A** Masking is rarely used in clinical hearing assessment
- [ ] **B** A 256-Hz tuning fork should ideally be used
- [ ] **C** A lateral Weber's test localisation may signify a conductive loss in that ear of at least 10 dB
- [ ] **D** Masking will correct a false-negative Rinne's test
- [ ] **E** Stenger's test is used to uncover feigned hearing loss

2.4 Regarding evoked response audiometry (ERA):

☐ **A** Electrocochleogram involves a needle placed through the eardrum on the promontory
☐ **B** Ménière's disease typically shows an increase in action potential
☐ **C** Patients need to be anaesthetised to undergo ERA
☐ **D** Brainstem electrical response audiometry (BERA) is the most sensitive test for acoustic neuroma
☐ **E** The BERA signal is made up of seven waves

2.5 Regarding hearing aids:

☐ **A** A quarter of octogenarians would benefit from hearing aids
☐ **B** Digital hearing aids are now widely available on the NHS
☐ **C** Bone conduction requires a direct connection between vibrator and skull
☐ **D** Bilateral hearing aids are recommended for bilateral deafness
☐ **E** The sound bridge is a new form of external hearing aid

2.6 Regarding impedance audiometry:

☐ **A** This involves altering compliance while pressure is measured
☐ **B** It may show a flat type C tympanogram
☐ **C** Maximum compliance occurs at minimum pressure difference
☐ **D** Presence of a stapedial reflex indicates an intact trigeminal nerve
☐ **E** Tympanometry can differentiate between otitis media with effusion and perforation

2.7 Non-organic hearing loss:

☐ **A** may be diagnosed using Stenger's test
☐ **B** is indicated by a stapedial reflex being < 20 dB above the reported pure tone threshold

2.8 When otoacoustic emissions (OAE) are measured:

☐ **A** An airtight seal with the external auditory meatus is required
☐ **B** Stimulus frequency emissions are the most useful clinically
☐ **C** The emissions originate in the outer hair cells
☐ **D** An anaesthetic is required

2.9 Presbyacusis:

☐ **A** is typically a low-frequency hearing loss
☐ **B** affects more than half of all 71–80-year-olds to at least a moderate degree
☐ **C** is treated with hearing aids in more than half of all sufferers

2.10 Regarding pure tone audiometry:

☐ **A** In a normal person a dB SPL (sound pressure level) audiogram should be flat
☐ **B** Testing involves increasing tones by increments of 5 dB
☐ **C** The Carhart effect is the artificial improvement of bone conduction thresholds by middle ear transmission
☐ **D** Masking frequencies should be close to the testing frequency

2.11 Sudden hearing loss:
- ☐ **A** is almost always sensorineural
- ☐ **B** will recover spontaneously in 60% of cases
- ☐ **C** is an indication for hospital admission if it occurs on one side
- ☐ **D** is treated effectively with steroids

2.12 Tinnitus:
- ☐ **A** is associated with a hearing loss at the same frequency
- ☐ **B** may indicate an acoustic neuroma
- ☐ **C** may be treated with a hearing aid
- ☐ **D** is associated with hyperacusis in about 40%

2.13 Regarding vertigo:
- ☐ **A** The semicircular canals contain otoconia
- ☐ **B** The vestibular system provides most of the information for balancing of the body
- ☐ **C** Hallpike's manoeuvre can be used to treat benign positional vertigo
- ☐ **D** Caloric testing is frequently used to test vestibular function

2.14 Conduction deafness is caused by:
- ☐ **A** Paget's disease of the bone
- ☐ **B** an acoustic neuroma
- ☐ **C** otosclerosis
- ☐ **D** a fracture through the petrous temporal bone
- ☐ **E** otitis media

3 OTOLOGY

3.1 Regarding cholesteatoma:
- ☐ **A** It is caused by a nest of non-keratinising squamous epithelium
- ☐ **B** It may result in a positive fistula test
- ☐ **C** A resulting deafness may be sensorineural or conductive
- ☐ **D** It may be congenital
- ☐ **E** It may be successfully treated by suction clearance

3.2 With regard to acute suppurative otitis media (ASOM):
- ☐ **A** It is most commonly caused by *Haemophilus influenzae*
- ☐ **B** Eustachian tube dysfunction is a risk factor
- ☐ **C** Peak incidence occurs between 7 and 13 years
- ☐ **D** Decongestants have been proved to have a role in treatment
- ☐ **E** Gradenigo's syndrome is a recognised complication

3.3 Concerning the complications of chronic suppurative otitis media (CSOM):
- [ ] **A** The risk of an intracranial abscess is around 1:100
- [ ] **B** A lateral sinus venous thrombosis is best investigated with CT scanning
- [ ] **C** Conservative antibiotic therapy should be avoided if intracranial pathology is suspected
- [ ] **D** Facial palsy in CSOM is usually secondary to a compression of the facial nerve

3.4 Regarding labyrinthitis:
- [ ] **A** In the Tullio phenomenon, loud sounds cause vertigo
- [ ] **B** In a labyrinthine fistula, the labyrinth endosteum is breached
- [ ] **C** A positive fistula sign on one side causes the patient to look towards that side
- [ ] **D** A patient with labyrinthitis will tend to look towards the affected side
- [ ] **E** A CT scan may be used to exclude a cerebral abscess

3.5 Mastoidectomy:
- [ ] **A** is necessary for inserting a cochlear implant
- [ ] **B** is the best treatment for a cholesteatoma when of the cortical type
- [ ] **C** is the best treatment for mastoiditis when of the cortical type
- [ ] **D** may preserve some hearing with apposition of the eardrum to the head of stapes
- [ ] **E** of the radical and cortical types are both performed in a combined-approach tympanoplasty

3.6 Ménière's disease:
- [ ] **A** classically consists of a triad of permanent vertigo, tinnitus, and hearing loss
- [ ] **B** classically shows a low-frequency hearing loss
- [ ] **C** is most common in the seventh decade
- [ ] **D** is exacerbated by the glycerol dehydration test
- [ ] **E** is due to an increase in endolymphatic fluid in the inner ear

3.7 Treatment of Ménière's disease:
- [ ] **A** Diet modification has been proved to be successful
- [ ] **B** Treatment by diuretics has been proved to be successful
- [ ] **C** Grommet insertion has been proved to be successful
- [ ] **D** Gentamicin application has been proved to be successful
- [ ] **E** Endolymphatic sac surgery has been proved to be successful

3.8 Regarding otalgia and the nerve supply of the ear:
- [ ] **A** The external ear is supplied by the facial nerve
- [ ] **B** The external ear is supplied by the greater auricular nerve inferiorly
- [ ] **C** The external ear is supplied by the mandibular nerve
- [ ] **D** The external auditory meatus is supplied by the vagus nerve
- [ ] **E** Jacobson's nerve originates from the vagus nerve
- [ ] **F** Alderman's nerve originates from the vagus nerve
- [ ] **G** Dental disease causes referred ear pain via the trigeminal nerve

3.9 Regarding otitis externa:
- ☐ **A** The outer two-thirds of the ear contains ceruminous glands
- ☐ **B** The pH of the ear is normally between 3 and 5
- ☐ **C** *Staphylococcus aureus* is a normal ear commensal
- ☐ **D** Malignant otitis externa is often caused by *Pseudomonas* infection
- ☐ **E** Aluminium acetate drops work by lowering pH
- ☐ **F** Mastoiditis characteristically causes upward displacement of the pinna

3.10 Regarding otitis media:
- ☐ **A** Swimming increases the risk of infection when grommets are in situ
- ☐ **B** T-tubes give rise to higher rates of residual perforation compared with Shah grommets
- ☐ **C** Tympanosclerosis is associated with extratympanic bleeding
- ☐ **D** Most cases of otitis media present between 6 and 12 years
- ☐ **E** Reduction in middle ear pressure draws in glue by pressure effects

3.11 Longitudinal fractures of the temporal bone:
- ☐ **A** are more likely to result in facial nerve injury than transverse fractures
- ☐ **B** commonly arise from a lateral skull blow
- ☐ **C** are more common than transverse fractures of the temporal bone
- ☐ **D** when accompanied by facial nerve weakness, are an indication for immediate exploration

3.12 Otosclerosis:
- ☐ **A** is an autosomal recessive condition
- ☐ **B** affects 0.2% of the population
- ☐ **C** is classically indicated by Schwartze's sign
- ☐ **D** has damage to the sense of taste as a recognised component
- ☐ **E** is bilateral in 85% of cases

3.13 In ototoxicity:
- ☐ **A** Gentamicin is largely vestibulotoxic
- ☐ **B** Neomycin is largely cochleotoxic
- ☐ **C** Susceptibility to aminoglycoside ototoxicity is X-linked
- ☐ **D** Loop diuretics may be ototoxic

3.14 A perilymph fistula:
- ☐ **A** may manifest itself as a sensorineural hearing loss
- ☐ **B** usually originates at the round window
- ☐ **C** is usually treated conservatively
- ☐ **D** may be congenital

3.15 Tympanoplasty:
- ☐ **A** involves the reconstruction of the hearing mechanism
- ☐ **B** may include eradication of middle ear disease
- ☐ **C** may include homografting
- ☐ **D** is a contraindication to diving

3.16 The chorda tympani:
- ☐ **A** contains taste fibres
- ☐ **B** is secretomotor to the parotid salivary gland
- ☐ **C** exits the middle ear via the stylomastoid foramen
- ☐ **D** is vulnerable to damage during parotid surgery
- ☐ **E** is damaged by compression at the stylomastoid foramen
- ☐ **F** joins the lingual nerve

3.17 Pain in the ear during acute tonsillitis is due to referral from the:
- ☐ **A** superior laryngeal nerve
- ☐ **B** glossopharyngeal nerve
- ☐ **C** facial nerve
- ☐ **D** hypoglossal nerve
- ☐ **E** lesser palatine nerve

3.18 Acute otitis media:
- ☐ **A** is often accompanied by a purulent discharge from the ear
- ☐ **B** is usually caused by *Escherichia coli*
- ☐ **C** rarely causes constitutional upset in children
- ☐ **D** invariably forms a cholesteatoma if resolution does not occur within 6 weeks
- ☐ **E** is primarily treated with myringotomy

3.19 Complications of otitis media include:
- ☐ **A** papilloedema
- ☐ **B** facial nerve paralysis
- ☐ **C** cerebellar abscess
- ☐ **D** homonymous hemianopia
- ☐ **E** sudden deafness

3.20 The middle ear:
- ☐ **A** has the facial nerve running through its roof
- ☐ **B** is lined with a mucous membrane
- ☐ **C** contains all the auditory ossicles
- ☐ **D** has the internal carotid artery running anteriorly
- ☐ **E** has a promontory in the projection of the lateral semicircular canal
- ☐ **F** has the internal jugular vein running medially

4 RHINOLOGY

4.1 Allergic rhinitis:
- ☐ **A** is commonly associated with polyps
- ☐ **B** involves attachment of the Fab portion of the IgE to the allergen
- ☐ **C** is an example of type II hypersensitivity
- ☐ **D** is often treated with long-term oral steroids
- ☐ **E** may be treated by surgical intervention

4.2 Epistaxis:

- ☐ **A** from the upper nose is commonly from the external carotid artery
- ☐ **B** may be treated by oestrogens in patients with hereditary haemorrhagic telangiectasia (HHT)
- ☐ **C** is idiopathic in most cases
- ☐ **D** may be treated by external carotid artery ligation
- ☐ **E** requires antibiotic cover if postnasal space packing is performed

4.3 Regarding granulomatous disease:

- ☐ **A** In cases of Wegener's granulomatosis (WG), p-ANCA s a sensitive test
- ☐ **B** WG is a necrotising vasculitis
- ☐ **C** Sarcoid is associated with non-caseating granulomas
- ☐ **D** WG is thought to have a bacterial precipitant
- ☐ **E** A renal biopsy is not necessary for the diagnosis of WG

4.4 Nasal polyps:

- ☐ **A** are commonly associated with asthma
- ☐ **B** are typically painful
- ☐ **C** are a sign of cystic fibrosis in childhood
- ☐ **D** are treated with long-term oral steroids
- ☐ **E** emerge from the ethmoid sinus when of the antrochoanal type

4.5 Nasal fractures:

- ☐ **A** may require open reduction
- ☐ **B** would raise concerns of CSF leak if accompanied by a clear rhinorrhoea
- ☐ **C** may be treated by simple aspiration if accompanied by a septal haematoma
- ☐ **D** show infraorbital nerve damage if accompanied by a numbness below the eye
- ☐ **E** should be treated conservatively for at least 2 weeks until the swelling has reduced

4.6 Regarding functional endoscopic sinus surgery (FESS):

- ☐ **A** Stripping of the nasal mucosa is usually necessary
- ☐ **B** Pituitary surgery may be performed by this method
- ☐ **C** A CSF leak should be repaired immediately
- ☐ **D** This is always performed front-to-back
- ☐ **E** Regular nasal douching is often part of postoperative care

4.7 Septal perforation:

- ☐ **A** usually affects the posterior cartilaginous system
- ☐ **B** may indicate the need for an ANCA test
- ☐ **C** is usually treated successfully with surgical closure
- ☐ **D** may be treated by enlargement of the perforation if it is causing whistling
- ☐ **E** may be caused by nose-picking

4.8 Regarding sinonasal tumours:

☐ **A** They are mostly adenocarcinomas
☐ **B** Working with wood is a risk factor for squamous cell carcinoma
☐ **C** Inverted papillomas may be treated endoscopically
☐ **D** They usually present relatively late
☐ **E** Lateral rhinostomy may be used for inverted papillomas

4.9 Sinusitis:

☐ **A** is associated with Kartagener's syndrome
☐ **B** in the acute form is most commonly due to *Staphylococcus aureus*
☐ **C** is usually treated with broad-spectrum antibiotics
☐ **D** is readily diagnosed by the finding of thickened mucosa on CT scanning
☐ **E** may be treated by removal of the entire sinus mucosa

4.10 Regarding smell and taste:

☐ **A** Olfaction is served by the trigeminal nerve
☐ **B** Gustation is served by the glossopharyngeal nerve
☐ **C** The tip of the tongue detects sour tastes
☐ **D** The posterior part of the tongue detects bitter tastes
☐ **E** Common chemical sensation mostly picks up unpleasant stimuli

4.11 Maxillary sinus carcinoma is associated with:

☐ **A** a chronic nasal foreign body
☐ **B** facial pain
☐ **C** trismus
☐ **D** enophthalmos
☐ **E** work in the hardwood industry
☐ **F** anosmia
☐ **G** proptosis

4.12 Epistaxis:

☐ **A** usually arises from the posteromedial nasal septum
☐ **B** can be controlled by placement of a Fogarty balloon catheter
☐ **C** may be a presentation of leukaemia
☐ **D** may require ligation of the maxillary artery
☐ **E** is best treated by bedrest and sedation

4.13 The nasopharynx:

☐ **A** receives a sensory supply from the glossopharyngeal nerve
☐ **B** contains the pharyngeal tonsil
☐ **C** is ridged by the palatopharyngeal fold
☐ **D** has the internal carotid artery lying against its wall
☐ **E** contains the pyramidal fossa
☐ **F** has a communication with the oropharynx that is closed during swallowing

4.14 Olfactory neuroblastoma:
- [ ] **A** frequently causes bilateral nasal obstruction
- [ ] **B** frequently presents with unilateral sinusitis symptoms
- [ ] **C** is a tumour of the neural crest stem cells
- [ ] **D** rarely involves the cribriform plate
- [ ] **E** can be resected via a craniofacial approach

5 LARYNGOLOGY

5.1 Concerning thyroglossal cysts:
- [ ] **A** More cysts lie on the left than on the right side
- [ ] **B** There is a role for radio-iodine scanning
- [ ] **C** They move with swallowing because they are attached to the hyoid
- [ ] **D** They may be confused on clinical examination with a dermoid cyst
- [ ] **E** Sistrunk's procedure includes excision of a wedge of hyoid bone
- [ ] **F** Recurrence after Sistrunk's procedure is 30%

5.2 Concerning branchial cysts:
- [ ] **A** They may arise from squamous epithelial remnants
- [ ] **B** 60% present on the right side
- [ ] **C** 60% present in men
- [ ] **D** 25% of cysts become infected
- [ ] **E** They lie posterior to the sternocleidomastoid muscle

5.3 Chemodectomas:
- [ ] **A** are more common at high altitude
- [ ] **B** should be biopsied by FNA
- [ ] **C** are best investigated by CT
- [ ] **D** may present as glomus jugulare tumours

5.4 Concerning cervical lymphadenopathy secondary to neoplasia:
- [ ] **A** Movable multiple ipsilateral nodes < 6 cm indicate an N2a tumour stage
- [ ] **B** In approximately 5–10% of cases the primary remains elusive
- [ ] **C** N1 nodes may be treated solely by radiotherapy
- [ ] **D** In N2 tumours, postoperative radiotherapy increases survival

5.5 Regarding cosmetic surgery:
- [ ] **A** It is important not to apply a tight head dressing post-pinnaplasty
- [ ] **B** Facial reanimation is not usually considered until 1 year after facial palsy onset
- [ ] **C** Facelifts involve elevation of the superficial muscle and aponeurotic system (SMAS)

5.6 Regarding facial nerve palsy:

- ☐ **A** It is usually due to Bell's palsy
- ☐ **B** It should be treated with low-dose steroids
- ☐ **C** It may be due to neoplasia
- ☐ **D** Lacrimation while eating is a poor prognostic sign
- ☐ **E** It is graded according to the Ramsay Hunt system

5.7 Concerning hypopharyngeal carcinoma:

- ☐ **A** Most tumours are adenocarcinoma
- ☐ **B** There is a strong association with tobacco and alcohol
- ☐ **C** There is an association with Plummer–Vinson–Patterson–Kelly syndrome (PVPK)
- ☐ **D** A tumour > 4 cm in diameter with no invasion of adjacent structures is a T3 tumour
- ☐ **E** Small tumours may be treated by watchful waiting
- ☐ **F** Patients rarely require calcium or thyroxine after surgery

5.8 Regarding laryngeal carcinoma:

- ☐ **A** Hoarseness is the most common feature
- ☐ **B** A fixed vocal cord indicates a T2 tumour
- ☐ **C** Glottic tumours metastasise early from extensive lymph drainage
- ☐ **D** A total laryngectomy usually includes a thyroidectomy

5.9 Nasopharyngeal carcinoma:

- ☐ **A** often involves the fossa of Rosenmuller
- ☐ **B** is associated with infectious mononucleosis
- ☐ **C** is often treated with surgery
- ☐ **D** typically affects young women in the case of angiofibromas
- ☐ **E** always involves the sphenopalatine foramen in the case of angiofibroma

5.10 A radical neck dissection:

- ☐ **A** may preserve the sternocleidomastoid muscle
- ☐ **B** should not be undertaken bilaterally
- ☐ **C** has frozen shoulder as a late complication
- ☐ **D** results in a 30-fold increase in intracranial pressure

5.11 Concerning neck space infections:

- ☐ **A** The parapharyngeal space extends from the skull base to the T3 vertebra
- ☐ **B** The styloid process divides the retropharyngeal space into anterior and posterior spaces
- ☐ **C** The infratemporal fossa is bounded superiorly by the petrous temporal bone
- ☐ **D** A parapharyngeal abscess is usually caused by tonsillitis
- ☐ **E** Submandibular abscesses are usually caused by tonsillitis
- ☐ **F** The posterior compartment of the parapharyngeal space contains the carotid artery

5.12 Concerning oral cavity carcinoma:
- [ ] **A** Most malignant tumours are adenocarcinomas
- [ ] **B** Alcohol consumption is a risk factor
- [ ] **C** The roof of the mouth is the commonest site
- [ ] **D** Neck nodes are only treated in T4 tumours
- [ ] **E** Both sides of the neck may need to be treated in a unilateral carcinoma

5.13 Regarding oropharyngeal carcinoma:
- [ ] **A** The anterior border of the oropharynx is the posterior tonsillar pillars
- [ ] **B** Non-Hodgkin's lymphoma (NHL) accounts for 50% of tumours
- [ ] **C** CT scanning is the best investigation

5.14 Regarding tracheostomy:
- [ ] **A** Decreasing dead space is not in itself an indication for tracheostomy
- [ ] **B** Some tracheostomy tubes are fenestrated to permit vocalisation
- [ ] **C** Paediatric tubes are usually non-cuffed
- [ ] **D** Percutaneous tracheostomy is cheaper than standard tracheostomy
- [ ] **E** The first change of tracheostomy tube should occur at 2 weeks

5.15 Regarding vocal cords:
- [ ] **A** Unilateral abduction palsy is treated by cord medialisation
- [ ] **B** Bilateral adductor palsy leads to aspiration
- [ ] **C** Recurrent laryngeal nerve supplies sensation below the vocal cords
- [ ] **D** Recurrent laryngeal nerve supplies the cricopharyngeus

5.16 Respiratory papillomatosis:
- [ ] **A** largely affects adults
- [ ] **B** is most effectively treated by surgery
- [ ] **C** carries a risk of malignant transformation

5.17 Pharyngeal pouches:
- [ ] **A** are usually anterior
- [ ] **B** arise from a defect in the middle constrictor muscle
- [ ] **C** arise from a defect between the thyropharyngeus and cricopharyngeus muscles
- [ ] **D** are best investigated with a CT scan
- [ ] **E** may be treated by endoscopic division
- [ ] **F** are often treated by thyropharyngeal myotomy

5.18 Regarding salivary glands:
- [ ] **A** Primary Sjögren's syndrome is associated with connective tissue disorders, eg rheumatoid arthritis
- [ ] **B** Papillary cystadenoma of the parotid gland is benign
- [ ] **C** Incisional biopsy is often necessary

5.19 Concerning salivary gland neoplasms:

- ☐ **A** They mostly originate in the parotid
- ☐ **B** They are 80% benign in the parotid
- ☐ **C** They are 50% benign in the minor salivary glands
- ☐ **D** They occur bilaterally in 50% of cases of Warthin's tumour
- ☐ **E** Adenocarcinoma is the most common malignant parotid tumour
- ☐ **F** Pleomorphic adenoma has a peak incidence in the seventh decade

5.20 Regarding obstructive sleep apnoea (OSA) and snoring:

- ☐ **A** OSA is defined as > 30 episodes of apnoea in 7 hours
- ☐ **B** OSA is always caused by airway obstruction
- ☐ **C** OSA affects 6% of men
- ☐ **D** 20% of men > 60 years suffer from snoring
- ☐ **E** OSA requiring CPAP is an indication for uvulopalatopharyngoplasty
- ☐ **F** OSA may require tracheostomy
- ☐ **G** Müller's manoeuvre may identify the site of obstruction

5.21 Regarding benign thyroid disease:

- ☐ **A** Graves' disease is associated with an IgA-mediated reaction
- ☐ **B** Hashimoto's thyroiditis is associated with hypothyroidism
- ☐ **C** The external branch of the superior laryngeal nerve is at risk in thyroid surgery
- ☐ **D** A 'cold' nodule is more likely to be malignant than a 'hot' one
- ☐ **E** Prendred's syndrome is associated with low-frequency hearing loss

5.22 Regarding malignant thyroid disease:

- ☐ **A** Follicular carcinoma is the most common
- ☐ **B** Papillary carcinoma spreads primarily via the bloodstream
- ☐ **C** FNA can accurately diagnose follicular adenocarcinoma
- ☐ **D** A subtotal thyroidectomy may be adequate treatment of papillary carcinoma
- ☐ **E** Medullary carcinoma is associated with multiple endocrine neoplasia (MEN) type 1

5.23 Tracheostomy:

- ☐ **A** may be complicated by tracheal stenosis
- ☐ **B** has to be formally closed after use
- ☐ **C** is a recognised cause of hypothyroidism
- ☐ **D** is best placed at the first tracheal cartilage
- ☐ **E** helps the cough reflex

5.24 Tracheostomy:

- ☐ **A** is uncomplicated by thyroid disease
- ☐ **B** may be needed for bronchial toilet
- ☐ **C** is straightforward in people with a short neck
- ☐ **D** will increase the anatomical dead space
- ☐ **E** increases the ventilation–perfusion mismatch

5.25 Papillary carcinoma of the thyroid:

☐ **A** commonly metastasises to the liver
☐ **B** is associated with endocrine tumours
☐ **C** is TSH-dependent
☐ **D** may present with hyperthyroidism
☐ **E** may be diagnosed by FNA cytology
☐ **F** is normally sensitive to radioactive iodine
☐ **G** should be treated with surgical resection if radioactive iodine treatment fails
☐ **H** has the best prognosis if the Hürthle-cell variant is present

5.26 Structures related to the superficial part of the submandibular gland include:

☐ **A** platysma
☐ **B** mandibular branch of the facial nerve
☐ **C** facial artery
☐ **D** facial vein
☐ **E** deep cervical fascia

5.27 Bilateral vocal cord paralysis:

☐ **A** is a recognised complication of diphtheria infection
☐ **B** may require intubation after thyroid surgery
☐ **C** is treated with arytenoidectomy
☐ **D** is caused by superior laryngeal nerve injury

5.28 Sjögren's syndrome:

☐ **A** is associated with rheumatoid arthritis
☐ **B** may follow a parotidectomy
☐ **C** is an autoimmune condition
☐ **D** causes lymphocyte infiltration in the parotid gland
☐ **E** causes dry eyes and dry mouth

6 PAEDIATRICS

6.1 With regard to adenoids:

☐ **A** Children with large adenoids commonly possess characteristic facies
☐ **B** A lateral soft tissue X-ray may give an indication of adenoid size
☐ **C** Cleft palate is an indication for adenoidectomy
☐ **D** Hypernasal speech is an indication for adenoidectomy

6.2 Choanal atresia:

☐ **A** usually presents as an emergency when bilateral
☐ **B** may be associated with an ear abnormality
☐ **C** is associated in 50% with facial nerve palsy
☐ **D** is associated in two-thirds with a laryngotracheal abnormality
☐ **E** often requires multiple redilations after being successfully repaired

6.3 In the case of chronic suppurative otitis media (CSOM):

☐ **A** A central perforation will more commonly lead to cholesteatoma than a peripheral one

☐ **B** A permanent perforation has a 40% chance of developing if a grommet has been in place for 2 years or more

☐ **C** A perforation usually leads to an air/bone conduction gap of > 30 dB

☐ **D** It more commonly leads to intracranial complications if cholesteatoma is present

☐ **E** Anaerobes are found in 50% of children with CSOM

6.4 With regard to cochlear implants and suitability for implantation:

☐ **A** They avoid the need for external devices

☐ **B** The ability to develop good speech requires hearing speech before the age of 6

☐ **C** Neural plasticity for audiological stimuli is lost around age 8

☐ **D** In adults, prelingual deafness is a contraindication to implantation

6.5 Common causes of unilateral nasal discharge include:

☐ **A** cystic fibrosis

☐ **B** nasal polyps

☐ **C** foreign body

☐ **D** common cold

☐ **E** nasopharyngeal carcinoma

6.6 Cleft lip:

☐ **A** affects boys more than girls

☐ **B** affects 1 in 750 live births

☐ **C** has a declining incidence

☐ **D** is associated with palate defects in 50% of cases

☐ **E** has a 25% subsequent increased risk if a previous child has been affected

6.7 Congenital hearing disorders:

☐ **A** are usually autosomal dominant

☐ **B** are usually sensorineural

☐ **C** are accompanied by a thyroid goitre in the case of Pendred's syndrome

☐ **D** may result from abnormalities of the first and second branchial arches

☐ **E** usually cause a conductive hearing loss in the case of rubella

6.8 Concerning epiglottitis:

☐ **A** It is usually caused by β-haemolytic streptococci

☐ **B** It is most common between the ages of 2 and 6 years

☐ **C** Its incidence has been reduced by 2-year olds receiving the Hib vaccine

☐ **D** The larynx/throat should be examined immediately

☐ **E** Chloramphenicol is an appropriate antibiotic

6.9 Foreign bodies:

☐ **A** may require a postaural incision if in the ear
☐ **B** may require an immediate barium swallow if in the throat
☐ **C** usually wedge at the thyropharyngeus if in the oesophagus
☐ **D** usually go down the right main bronchus, if in the bronchi
☐ **E** in the throat can be excluded on the basis of a clear lateral neck X-ray alone

6.10 Regarding paediatric airway problems:

☐ **A** Stertor originates in the larynx
☐ **B** Stridor, if inspiratory, is most likely to originate from the larynx
☐ **C** Subglottic stenosis may require reconstruction of the airway
☐ **D** Stridor may indicate abnormal blood vessel anatomy

6.11 Concerning paediatric hearing tests:

☐ **A** Preschool children aged 4–5 years may be tested with pure tone audiometry
☐ **B** Otoacoustic emission screening is routinely performed on children
☐ **C** Conditional reflex testing is performed with the child asleep
☐ **D** Evoked response audiometry is performed with the child awake
☐ **E** It is not possible to provide an objective test of hearing in a child under 3 months old

6.12 Tonsillitis:

☐ **A** is known to be due to bacterial infection
☐ **B** should be treated with amoxicillin as a first-line treatment
☐ **C** in cases referred to hospital, a Paul–Bunnell test is usually indicated
☐ **D** is known as quinsy if accompanied by a retropharyngeal abscess
☐ **E** may be associated with an acute glomerulonephritis

6.13 Tonsillectomy:

☐ **A** is indicated if a child is having tonsillitis twice a year
☐ **B** leads to postoperative haemorrhage in 10% of cases
☐ **C** may require suturing of the faucial pillars in intractable secondary bleeding
☐ **D** can cause bleeding, most likely from the tonsillar branch of the facial artery
☐ **E** may affect the voice quality

6.14 The following anatomical differences in children may make management of their airway more difficult than in adults:

☐ **A** A more caudally placed larynx
☐ **B** Smaller angle of the jaw
☐ **C** A more U-shaped epiglottis
☐ **D** A relatively large tongue
☐ **E** A larger head size compared with the body size

6.15 Glue ear is associated with:

- ☐ **A** enlarged pharyngeal tonsils
- ☐ **B** cleft palate
- ☐ **C** eustachian tube dysfunction
- ☐ **D** otosclerosis

6.16 The eustachian tube in the infant:

- ☐ **A** connects the middle ear to the oropharynx
- ☐ **B** opens by the palatine tonsil
- ☐ **C** has a bony portion in the sphenoid bone
- ☐ **D** has a cartilaginous medial segment
- ☐ **E** is more horizontal in the child

6.17 In a 10-year-old child with an 11-month history of a midline swelling just below the hyoid bone:

- ☐ **A** A Trucut biopsy is a useful test
- ☐ **B** The swelling is most likely to be a thyroglossal cyst
- ☐ **C** An ultrasound scan is the most useful first-line test
- ☐ **D** A technetium scan is useful
- ☐ **E** The swelling will resolve spontaneously

6.18 Recognised complications of acute tonsillitis include:

- ☐ **A** cholesteatoma
- ☐ **B** acute glomerulonephritis
- ☐ **C** quinsy
- ☐ **D** endotoxaemia
- ☐ **E** vocal cord palsy

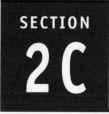

SECTION

2C Answers

CONTENTS

Extended Matching Questions (EMQs) – Answers

1 BASIC SCIENCE

1.1 Peripheral nerve anatomy

1 B   Lingual nerve

The lingual nerve serves proprioception to the muscles of the tongue, as well as general sensation to the mucous membrane over the anterior two-thirds of the tongue (taste is from the chorda tympani nerve – VII). It can be damaged in dental extraction by misapplication of dental forceps.

2 A   Facial nerve

Facial paralysis often goes unnoticed by patients with Bell's palsy. However, other ipsilateral symptoms may cause concern, including dry eye (loss of lacrimal sensation), leading to corneal ulceration and impaired vision; some loss of taste (from the anterior two-thirds of the tongue); inability to close the mouth, and the collection of food in the vestibule (paralysis of the buccinator muscle). This particular lesion is located in the nerve at or before the origin of the superior petrosal branch.

3 C   Ophthalmic nerve

In herpes zoster infection of the ophthalmic branch of cranial nerve V, a rash appears over the forehead from the vertex to the upper eyelid, extending over the ala of the nose (the external branch of the nasociliary nerve). If the cornea is involved (ciliary branch), blindness may result from scarring.

1.2 Selection of drains for surgical procedures

1 C   Suction

The traditional view is that a suction drain is needed after thyroid or parathyroid surgery, as haematoma can lead to rapid airway compromise.

2 B or D   Corrugated or tube drain

It is usual to leave a drain in situ to prevent further collection of haematoma, which could compromise the blood supply to the ear cartilage.

3 C   Suction

A suction drain prevents any build-up of haematoma and assists close adherence of the neck flaps. It can be removed when output is minimal.

4 E   None

No potential spaces exist for accumulation of blood and therefore no drain is required.

1.3 Nutrition

1 A   Nasogastric feeding

If possible, nutrition should be administered enterally, as continued functioning of the gastrointestinal system has been shown to have many benefits to the health of the patient. Insertion of a nasogastric tube will have no deleterious effect on the patient, and is the simplest solution for short-term nutritional supplementation.

2 B   Jejunostomy feeding

A feeding jejunostomy is a popular route for feeding after major oesophageal operations. The use of special feeds containing glutamine, for example, is gaining popularity but is not yet widely accepted.

1.4 Consent for surgical treatment

1 A   Yes, surgery can proceed

Surgery is needed for the preservation of life and can be performed despite the patient's inability to give consent. The patient's wife cannot give permission or stop her husband's operation. No adult can act as legal proxy for any other in the UK with regard to giving consent for surgical treatment.

2 C   Apply to make the child a ward of court

The surgeon can either respect the patient's wishes and not subject the child to an operation, or can make an application for the child to be made a ward of court and proceed with appropriate surgical treatment. In this case, surgical treatment is essential and almost all surgeons would go for the latter option.

3 A   Yes, surgery can proceed

The current Mental Health Act does not allow for the compulsory treatment of any condition other than a mental disorder. The ENT surgeon may, however, proceed with surgery for the patient's dysphagia if the surgeon and psychiatrist agree that it is the best form of management for her. It is good clinical practice also to obtain a second consultant surgical opinion confirming the need for operative treatment and to involve the relatives in the decision-making process where possible. Every clinician should make detailed entries in the patient's records and sign and date them.

4 B   No, surgery cannot proceed

Before the deterioration of this patient's condition he clearly refused to give consent for operative treatment. Surgery therefore cannot be performed even when his wife considers this to be an essential intervention.

1.5 Micro-organisms

1 B   *Streptococcus pneumoniae*

Ludwig's angina is bilateral infection of the submandibular, sublingual and submental spaces, usually arising from dental sepsis. Streptococcal infection spreads in deep cervical and pharyngeal fascial planes. It may cause airway obstruction.

2 G   None of the above

Vincent's angina is due to the symbiotic action of fusiform bacteria and the spirochaete *Borrelia vincentii*. It is a pharyngeal infection with ulcerative gingivitis.

3 C   *Clostridium difficile*

Following broad-spectrum antibiotic treatment, infection with *Clostridium difficile* may lead to pseudomembranous colitis.

1.6 Anticoagulant treatment regimens

1 D   Tinzaparin 3500 U once daily

Heparin is used in the prophylaxis and treatment of venous thrombosis and in the maintenance of anticoagulation in patients on warfarin who require surgery. For treatment and prophylaxis of thrombosis, the choice lies between unfractionated and low molecular weight heparin (LMWH), eg tinzaparin. Options B and D would provide comparable thromboprophylaxis, but there is evidence that LMWH is associated with less bleeding and is therefore preferable. LMWH also only requires once-daily injection and no routine monitoring of coagulation.

2 E   Tinzaparin 175 U once daily

This patient should be treated for a confirmed venous thrombosis and either unfractionated heparin or LMWH would be justified here. However, the APTT ratio target quoted in option C should be 1.5–2.5.

3 C   Unfractionated heparin iv to maintain an APTT ratio of 2.5–3.5

The patient requires conversion to heparin to enable rapid changes to be made to his level of anticoagulation perioperatively. Although LMWHs show more predictable bioavailability than unfractionated heparins, they have a longer half-life and laboratory monitoring is less straightforward. Because the level of anticoagulation is critical in this patient, most haematologists would advocate using unfractionated heparin to maintain an APTT of 2.5–3.5.

1.7 Treatment of bleeding in an anticoagulated patient

1 D   Vitamin K iv and fresh frozen plasma 30 ml/kg
This is a common problem where a patient who has been stable on warfarin for many years becomes over-anticoagulated because antibiotics have impaired hepatic metabolism of warfarin. Life-threatening bleeding is treated with a slow iv infusion of 5 mg phyto-menadione (vitamin K) and fresh frozen plasma. Vitamin K im should be avoided as it has poor bioavailability and is likely to cause a haematoma. Less severe haemorrhage may require 0.5–2 mg vitamin K iv and withdrawal of warfarin until the INR returns to the normal range. Elevation of the INR without bleeding may just require cessation of anti-coagulation and observation.

2 F   Protamine sulphate iv
This patient requires urgent heparin neutralisation with iv protamine sulphate (maximum 50 mg). Since the half-life of heparin is short, less severe bleeding may be safely treated by cessation of heparin and observation.

1.8 Suture materials

1 A   Absorbable, braided, synthetic

2 D   Non-absorbable, monofilament, synthetic

3 B   Absorbable, monofilament, synthetic

4 D   Non-absorbable, monofilament, synthetic

5 B   Absorbable, monofilament, synthetic

6 A   Absorbable, braided, synthetic

7 C   Non-absorbable, braided, natural material

2 AUDIOLOGY

2.1 Conditions

1 A   Ménière's disease
The episodic nature is important in the diagnosis; fullness in the ear may be present as a pre-attack symptom.

2 D   Noise-induced hearing loss
Often tinnitus is present at this frequency.

3 E   Acoustic neuroma
Vertigo and unsteadiness may be late symptoms.

2.2 Audiological/vestibular tests – 1

1 G   Tympanometry

2 E   Caloric testing
This is the best vestibular test for testing each side separately.

3 D   Brainstem electrical response audiometry

2.3 Audiological/vestibular tests – 2

1 F   Stenger's test
The fact that someone with bilateral hearing will hear only the loudest of two identical-pitch tuning forks is used in this test.

2 H   Unterberger's test
This is a test of the vestibulospinal reflex.

3 D   Weber's test

4 G   Bing test

2.4 Diagnoses

1 B   Left-sided conductive deafness

2 D   Left-sided sensorineural hearing loss

3 G   Normal hearing

2.5 Audiological aids

1 B   Bone-anchored hearing aid
Hearing aids may be difficult to fit.

2 F   Cooksey–Cawthorne exercises

3 G   Epley manoeuvre
She is most likely to be suffering from benign positional vertigo.

2.6 Audiovestibular structures

1 B   Superior vestibular nerve

2 G   Outer hair cell mechanism
The outer hair cells are thought to perform a motor as well as a sensory function, and are hence the site of the generation of otoacoustic emissions.

3 D   Medial geniculate body
The nerve then proceeds to the cerebral cortex.

4 A   Cochlear nerve
So it lies in front of the two vestibular nerves, which pierce the posterior quadrants of the temporal bone.

2.7 Vertigo

1 F   Labyrinthitis
Labyrinthitis is thought to be due to viral infection and may follow an upper respiratory tract infection. Treatment is symptomatic.

2 G   Benign paroxysmal positional vertigo
Treatment is symptomatic in acute phases, and vestibular exercises may help the vestibular system to readjust itself.

3 C   Cerebrovascular ischaemia
Ischaemia of the vestibular system may accompany other neurological symptoms or may be an isolated problem.

4 D   Ménière's disease
Attacks due to Ménière's disease usually last less than an hour and are accompanied by tinnitus and nausea. There is often a prodromal phase, usually involving a sensation of heaviness in the affected ear.

5 A   Application of cold water to right ear
Application of cold water to the ear during caloric testing causes nystagmus to the contralateral side, whereas application of hot water causes nystagmus to the same side.

3   OTOLOGY

3.1 Anatomy

1 A   Greater auricular nerve
Made up of C2 and C3, a branch of the cervical plexus.

2 C   Jacobson's nerve
Also known as the lesser petrosal nerve (tympanic branch of the glossopharyngeal nerve).

3 B   Alderman's/Arnold's nerve
A branch of vagus nerve.

3.2 Micro-organisms

1 A   *Streptococcus pneumoniae*
This is acute otitis media, a bacterial disease caused by pus-forming organisms. *S. pneumoniae* is the most likely cause (40%) followed by *H. influenzae* (30%).

2 D   *Pseudomonas* spp.
This is malignant otitis externa.

3 F   Epstein–Barr virus
Also known as glandular fever.

3.3 Antibiotics

1 B   Penicillin
Not augmentin as this may be glandular fever.

2 G   Gentamicin
In the form of eardrops.

3 A   Augmentin
Best coverage of ASOM (acute suppurative otitis media) pathogens.

3.4 Chronic suppurative otitis media

1 G   Gradenigo's syndrome
Associated with petrositis of the temporal bone.

2 F   Tympanosclerosis
A large plaque is needed to cause measurable hearing loss.

3 H   Labyrinthitis

3.5 Embryology

1 A   First pharyngeal arch

2 C   Second pharyngeal arch

3 B   First pharyngeal pouch

4 G   Sixth pharyngeal pouch

3.6 Temporal bone

1 C   Stylomastoid foramen

2 A   Squamous temporal bone

3 B   Petrous temporal bone

4 D   Tympanic plate of temporal bone

3.7 Pathology

1 A   Tullio phenomenon
May be secondary to Ménière's disease or to a fistula.

2 D   Hitselberger sign
This is a sign of an acoustic neuroma affecting other cranial nerves, in this case the vagus.

3 E   Schwartze's sign
In otosclerosis, 10% of ears show this sign; caused by dilated vessels on the promontory of the mucous membrane.

3.8 Middle ear nerves

1 B   Tympanic nerve

2 E   Lesser petrosal nerve

3 D   Chorda tympani

3.9 Diagnoses

1 J   Wax
Wax has narrowed the ear canal, which is then suddenly obstructed by a minimal amount of water that causes the wax to swell.

2 H   Otitis externa
Otitis externa is most commonly caused by scratching or inappropriate cleaning.

3 F   Chronic serous otitis media
Middle ear effusions are caused by blockage of the eustachian tube, whether this be by acute respiratory tract infections leading to acute otitis media, or by chronic obstructions such as sinusitis or, as in this case, a nasopharyngeal carcinoma.

4 E   Cholesteatoma
Cholesteatoma requires aggressive treatment, often including mastoidectomy, and has numerous extra- and intracranial complications.

5 I   Otosclerosis
Otosclerosis affects 1 in 200 people to some degree. It is more common in women and is hereditary to some degree. It commonly presents between the ages of 18 and 30, and tends to worsen during pregnancy. There is excessive bone formation in the middle ear leading to conductive deafness. Hearing is often improved in noisy places – so-called Willis' paracusis.

6 A   Acoustic neuroma
Around 80% of cerebellopontine angle tumours and 8% of intracranial tumours are acoustic neuromas. They arise from the neurilemmal cells of cranial nerves, usually in the internal auditory meatus. The tumour is benign but causes pressure effects on other cranial nerves (V, VII and others). Acoustic neuroma should be suspected in cases of unilateral deafness or tinnitus.

4 RHINOLOGY

4.1 Anatomy

1 A   Ethmoidal bone

2 F   Vomer

3 H   Frontal bone

4.2 Epistaxis

1 B   Hereditary haemorrhagic telangiectasia
This is also known as Osler–Weber–Rendu syndrome.

2 D   Angiofibroma
Most common between the ages of 10 and 25, most will resolve spontaneously.

3 G   Liver failure
Leading to a clotting disorder.

4.3 Arteries

1 B   Sphenopalatine artery
A branch of the maxillary artery from the external carotid artery.

2 D   Anterior ethmoidal artery
From the internal carotid artery.

2 C   Superior labial artery
Supplies anterior inferior region, from the facial artery.

4.4 Imaging techniques

1 A   CT scan
Although it is not appropriate to proceed to a CT scan until medical therapy has been trialed.

2 A   CT scan

3 G   Barium swallow

4 D   Plain X-ray
To investigate for lung pathology.

4.5 Diagnoses

1 C   Intrinsic rhinitis

2 D   Rhinitis medicamentosa

3 A   Antrochoanal polyp
The polyp acts as a ball valve, and blocks the eustachian tube.

4.6 Interventions

1 B   Septorhinoplasty

2 F   Conservative medical treatment
This may be sinusitis, but medical treatment is warranted before a CT scan is carried out.

3 D   Polypectomy

4.7 Taste sensation

1 E   Foliate papillae
Foliate papillae lie on the posterior lateral portion of the anterior two-thirds of the tongue.

2 F   Fungiform papillae
Fungiform papillae lie at the front of the tongue and detect sweet and salt taste.

3 D   Trigeminal nerve
Chemical sensation is often confused with true taste, and represents a direct chemical stimulation of the sensory nerve. As well as the trigeminal, the glossopharyngeal and vagus nerves may also be involved.

4.8 Relations

1 D   Frontal sinus
The frontal sinuses are related posteriorly to the frontal lobe of the brain and drain inferiorly into the anterior end of the hiatus semilunaris.

2 F   Maxillary sinus
The maxillary sinus projects into the zygomatic process of the temporal bone, and is related posteriorly to the infratemporal fossa and pterygopalatine fossa. It is grooved superiorly by the infraorbital nerve, and drains into the hiatus semilunaris.

3 B   Ethmoid sinus
The ethmoidal air cells and grouped into anterior (opening into the hiatus semilunaris), middle (within the bulla ethmoidalis), and posterior (draining into the superior meatus).

4 H   Sphenoid sinus
The sphenoid sinus in the body of the sphenoid bone forms the sella turcica. It drains into the spheno-ethmoidal recess.

5 E   Inferior concha
The nasolacrimal duct lies between the maxillary laterally and the lacrimal and inferior conchal bones medially. The nasal opening is overlain by a fold of mucosa.

4.9 Diagnoses

1 C   Foreign body
Foreign body insertion is commonest at the age of 2–3.

2 D   Leukaemia
Leukaemia and other blood dyscrasias may present with epistaxis as a result of clotting abnormalities caused by thrombocytopenia.

3 B   Drug-induced
Warfarin levels may make treatment of epistaxis problematic.

4 G   Pyogenic granuloma
Pyogenic granulomas are smooth red swellings that arise most frequently in Little's area. They may cause severe bleeding and may mimic a neoplasm. They can generally be easily removed under GA.

5 F   Osler–Weber–Rendu disease
Osler–Weber–Rendu disease, or hereditary haemorrhagic telangiectasia, can give rise to severe and occasionally fatal haemorrhage. Many treatments have been tried, including sclerosants, split-skin grafting, ligation, or embolisation of the feeding vessels.

5 LARYNGOLOGY

5.1 Nerve damage

1 F   Accessory nerve
Always damaged in radical neck dissections.

2 A   Recurrent laryngeal nerve
Probably a unilateral adductor palsy.

3 H   Hypoglossal nerve
The hypoglossal nerve controls intrinsic tongue muscles and runs near to the submandibular duct capsule.

5.2 Foramina

1 C   Foramen rotundum

2 G   Jugular foramen

3 I   Foramen magnum

5.3 Muscles

1 D   Tensor veli palati

2 B   Palatopharyngeus

3 I   Hyoglossus

5.4 Histological diagnoses

1 A   Adenocarcinoma
Nasosinal adenocarcinoma associated with hardwood dust.

2 C   Mucoepidermoid carcinoma
The commonest malignant parotid tumour.

3 G   Pleomorphic adenoma

5.5 Facial nerve palsy

1 C   Ramsay Hunt syndrome

2 G   Multiple sclerosis

3 B   Bell's palsy

5.6 Neck lumps

1 B   Chemodectoma
Living at a high altitude is a risk factor.

2 C   Branchial cyst

3 E   Thyroglossal cyst

5.7 Thyroid neoplasms

1 D   Medullary carcinoma
MEN 2, with a previous phaeochromocytoma.

2 C   Papillary adenoma
Commonest cause of papillary carcinoma.

3 E   Anaplastic carcinoma
This carries a very poor prognosis.

5.8 Surgical complications

1 A   Superficial parotidectomy
Gustatory sweating.

2 F   Functional endoscopic sinus surgery
Perforation of the lamina papyracea is a risk.

3 B   Radical neck dissection
An inevitable consequence.

4 A   Superficial parotidectomy
Damage to the facial nerve, which often recovers.

5.9 Thyroid cancer

1 D   Anaplastic carcinoma
Anaplastic carcinoma has one of the worst prognoses of thyroid carcinomas. It is a very aggressive tumour, invading all local structures early.

2 E   Lymphoma
Lymphoma responds very well to radiotherapy and this may be the only treatment necessary after a diagnostic biopsy has been taken.

3 A   Papillary carcinoma
Papillary carcinoma of the thyroid is four times more common in women. It tends to affect young people, is multicentric and metastasises early to lymph nodes.

4 C   Medullary cell carcinoma
Medullary thyroid carcinoma is sporadic in 90% of cases. Familial cases may be associated with MEN 2. Calcitonin is a good tumour marker for medullary thyroid cancer because it is known to be secreted from parafollicular C cells.

5 B   Follicular carcinoma
Follicular carcinoma of the thyroid tends to be solitary, encapsulated, invading the bloodstream and spreading to bone.

6 PAEDIATRICS

6.1 Airway difficulty

1 C   Choanal atresia
Choanal atresia usually presents very soon after birth and is often accompanied by feeding difficulties. An investigation for the CHARGE syndrome should be conducted.

2 E   Subglottic stenosis
A laryngotracheal reconstruction procedure may be required to provide permanent relief from airway difficulties.

3 D   Laryngomalacia
No treatment is indicated if the airway difficulty is not life-threatening.

6.2 Airway interventions

1 B   Laryngotracheal reconstruction
Reconstruction may be achieved by using costal cartilage to stent the stenotic airway open.

2 A   Nasal prong
Anatomical arrangement of the nasal airway in Pierre Robin syndrome produces chronic stertor – bilateral nasal prongs will keep the airway open.

3 C   Tonsillectomy
This would be the simplest way of improving breathing.

6.3 Hearing tests

1 D   Auditory response cradle
The auditory response cradle monitors four behavioural responses to sound – head turning, startle responses, body movements and respiratory changes. Otoacoustic responses might also be appropriate in this case.

2 A   Distraction testing
This is the standard screening test for children of this age.

3 C   Electrocochleogram
The electrocochleogram is the only way of assessing specific frequencies objectively.

6.4 Interventions

1 A   Adenoidectomy
With no chronic effusion present, grommets will provide no benefit.

2 C   Shah grommet insertion
Cleft palate is a contraindication for adenotonsillectomy. Children with cleft palates also often suffer with glue ear, and often grommets are inserted prophylactically.

3 E   No surgical intervention needed
The frequency of tonsillitis is not enough to justify operative intervention at this stage – at least four episodes per year for at least 2 years is the commonly accepted criterion.

6.5 Diagnoses

1 A   Epiglottitis
Epiglottitis is declining in incidence due to the influence of the Hib vaccine. It is a medical emergency, and a child should not be examined to avoid further compromising the airway. Anaesthetic assistance should be sought and intubation achieved as soon as possible – treatment is with intravenous antibiotics.

2 E   Laryngomalacia
Stridor will improve with time, and no operative intervention is indicated.

3 D   Papillomata
Laryngeal papillomatosis is treated with regular laser surgery until the child eventually grows out of the condition.

6.6 Congenital hearing disorders

1 D   Apert's syndrome

2 A   Pendred's syndrome

3 F   Mondini dysplasia

6.7 Age at diagnosis

1 A At birth
This requires urgent surgical correction, as newborn babies are obligate nasal breathers.

2 B In the first year of life
Subglottic stenosis usually develops after prolonged intubation secondary to prematurity, and presents after extubation.

3 C Between 2 and 5
Although an effusion may develop from birth, its effects are not usually diagnosed until the child is a few years old. Incidence of glue ear decreases as the child gets older.

Multiple True/False Questions – Answers

1 BASIC SCIENCES

1.1 AB

Investigations indicated preoperatively will vary from centre to centre, but people with asthma usually need a chest X-ray only if there is some reason to believe that their disease status has deteriorated since the last investigation. ECGs are usually indicated only for those over 60 or for those with cardiac symptoms.

Nitrous oxide is a common anaesthetic, and is easily soluble in blood, leading to its diffusion into air-containing spaces such as the middle ear – it has been noted by some surgeons that use of nitrous oxide exerts some internal pressure on a newly-laid tympanic membrane graft, so aiding positioning. In general, the gases used in anaesthesia are, as with most surgery, flammable, and care must be taken when laser therapy is used to avoid causing an airway fire.

The laryngeal mask airway consists of a cuffed tube that sits at the entrance to the larynx. As such it does not directly intubate the trachea, and is therefore to be viewed as a temporary measure, pending the establishment of a secure airway.

1.2 E

Local anaesthetics work better at higher pH, when they are less ionised. Infected tissue has an increased blood supply, which could lead to rapid absorption and hazardous effects – hence a general anaesthetic may be a better choice. Bupivacaine lasts longer than prilocaine, which in turn lasts longer than lidocaine; the safe dosages of lidocaine are 3 mg/kg, or 7 mg/kg with adrenaline.

Moffett's solution is a cocktail of anaesthetic agents, used commonly in the pre-operative anaesthesia of nasal polyps before removal. There are many variations but the classic recipe is 2 ml of 8–10% cocaine, 1 ml of 1:1000 adrenaline and 2 ml of 1% sodium bicarbonate, sprayed on both sides to cover the anterior compartment mucous membranes of the nose.

1.3 All true

Laser is an acronym for light amplification by stimulated emission of radiation. The light produced is monochromatic, parallel and in-phase. It may be passed through a lens for focusing. The CO_2 laser is accurate with not much penetration, and is most commonly used for throat lesions. The NdYAG laser is used in fibreoptic work, and provides coagulation at the same time as cutting. The potassium titanyl phosphate (KTP) laser is used in the excision of deeper lesions that are more likely to bleed, and also in the ear and nose. The argon laser is well absorbed by blood and accurate, and so will be of use around small vessels. When using a laser, all staff should wear eye protection, and the theatre should be fitted with an automatic lock and alarm system.

1.4 ABE

Consent is either implied (for example by undressing before being examined) or explicit (as obtained before operations). Risks that the patient is likely to attach significance to should be explained, but the principle of therapeutic privilege means that a doctor may choose to withhold some information if he feels it would not be in the patient's interests.

Negligence claims must prove harm to the patient to be successful. The Bowlam test states that a doctor is not guilty of negligence if he acts in accordance with the practice of a responsible body of medical people. Perioperative dental damage is the most common cause of ENT litigation.

1.5 CE

T1 MRI images provide best pictures of soft tissue, whereas T2 gives better contrast for the detection of abnormal tissue. Lateral soft tissue X-rays are not essential for suspected foreign bodies – it is better to rely on the clinical symptoms.

In the case of swallow investigations, water-soluble agents should be used if aspiration of leakage is a possibility.

Sinusitis should not be diagnosed via CT scan – rather, the scans should be used as an aid to subsequent surgery. Chest X-ray in the case of a sudden unexplained laryngeal nerve palsy may show a lung neoplasm.

1.6 AC

During exercise cardiac output increases sixfold (heart rate $\times$ 3 and stroke volume $\times$ 2). There is usually no change in PaO_2 and $PaCO_2$. An increase in systolic and a decrease in diastolic pressure are seen. Renal blood flow is reduced and there is an increase in negative intrathoracic pressure.

1.7 BC

Men > 50 should have an ECG as their incidence of ischaemic heart disease is higher than in those < 50. Smokers should have a chest X-ray as they may have concurrent cardiac problems, pneumonia or carcinoma of the lung. Consent is obtained when the patient is of sound mind, can make a balanced informed decision and can understand the information. Premedication often contains benzodiazepines, which cause drowsiness and impair concentration and cognition.

1.8 DE

Pulse oximeters monitor pulse rate, pulse volume and oxygen saturation. The oxygen saturation can be normal from a high inspired oxygen level. Pulse oximetry is accurate to 2%. Pulse amplitude is only an indicator of cardiac output. A high concentration of carboxyhaemoglobin can cause a pulse oximeter to give a falsely elevated reading. All colour changes are sensed. The change in path length caused by arterial pulsation allows for the subtraction of changes caused by capillary and venous blood.

1.9 CDE

Monopolar diathermy uses an alternating current as a frequency of 400 kHz–10 MHz. Current passes down the diathermy forceps, which may be applied to surgical forceps holding tissue, causing a local heating effect (up to 1000 °C) through the patient plate electrode (which must be at least 70 cm^2 in size). Bipolar diathermy avoids the need for the patient plate, and it uses less power as the current passes down one limb of the forceps and back up the other. Bipolar diathermy may be applied through surgical forceps and cannot be used for cutting tissue. Monopolar diathermy may be used in patients with a pacemaker, but should be used in short bursts of less than 2 seconds and the diathermy circuit should be away from the site of the pacemaker. It is preferable to use bipolar diathermy in these patients. Diathermy burns are usually full-thickness.

1.10 D

Body water content is 60% in the adult man and this equates to about 45 litres. (Neonates comprise 75% water.) The plasma volume measures about 3.5 litres and the total blood volume is about 5 litres. Approximately 400 ml of water is lost daily from the lungs. The intracellular fluid is about two-thirds of total body water, ie 30 litres out of 45 litres. Daily potassium requirements are roughly 1 mmol/kg. The normal serum potassium concentration is about 3.5–5.0 mmol/kg.

1.11 BD

Cytology does not give architectural histology. Gram staining is not part of the FNAC. FNAC can be used to diagnose thyroid lumps but cannot distinguish between follicular adenoma and follicular carcinoma.

1.12 BDE

Laboratory features of iron deficiency anaemia include: decreased serum iron concentration; a raised TIBC; and absent iron in both the marrow and erythroblasts. Tissue oxygen delivery is dependent on haemoglobin and therefore will be affected. Anaemia does not cause a shift in the oxygen dissociation curve. The presence of a posterior cricoid web and iron deficiency is a recognised association (Plummer–Vinson–Patterson–Kelly syndrome). Treatment with aspirin can cause gastritis, and associated haemoglobin loss over a prolonged period can deplete iron stores.

1.13 AF

Coagulation is initiated in vivo by the exposure of circulating factor VII to tissue factor, which in turn activates factor X (extrinsic pathway). Activated factor X subsequently sustains and amplifies the pathway by activating more factor VII and by activating factors XII, XI, IX, VIII and V (intrinsic pathway). Both pathways generate more activated factor, which, in sufficient concentration, converts prothrombin to thrombin – this in turn converts fibrinogen to fibrin (common pathway) so producing a fibrin clot. The process is complemented by factor XIII, which stabilises the fibrin clot. Clotting factors are predominantly synthesised in the liver, factors II, VII, IX and X synthesis being vitamin K-dependent. The coagulation cascade is inhibited in vivo by antithrombin III and the protein S and C pathways, hence deficiency of these proteins predisposes to thrombosis. Deficiency of the extrinsic, intrinsic and common pathway factors predisposes to haemorrhage, with the exception of factor XII deficiency, which is asymptomatic.

1.14 AC

The foramen spinosum transmits the middle meningeal vessels and the meningeal branch of the mandibular nerve. The foramen rotundum contains the maxillary nerve. The foramen ovale transmits the mandibular nerve, lesser petrosal nerve and accessory meningeal artery. The foramen lacerum transmits the internal carotid and greater petrosal nerve, which leaves as a nerve of the pterygoid canal.

1.15 CE

The recurrent laryngeal nerve supplies all the intrinsic muscles of the larynx except the cricothyroid and is sensory inferior to the vocal folds. In the neck, the recurrent laryngeal nerves on both sides follow the same course, ascending in the tracheo-oesophageal groove. As the nerve passes the lateral lobe of the thyroid, it is closely related to the inferior thyroid artery. The superior laryngeal nerve supplies the vocal cord mucosa.

1.16 CE

Audit is defined as 'the systemic, clinical analysis of the quality of medical care, including the procedures used for diagnosis and treatment, the use of resources, and the resulting outcome and quality of life for the patient'. There are three main elements to audit:

- **Structure** refers to the available patient resources.
- **Process** is what is done to the patient.
- **Outcome** is the result of the clinical intervention.

Audit does not only concern doctors, but also other healthcare professionals. It can be consultant-led, but individual practices vary. Standards are ideally set by a multidisciplinary team. While audit aims to improve the quality of patient care, its prime interest is in whether standards have been met and not outcome analysis (which is better served by controlled ratios).

1.17 ABF

A moral right is one that an individual can claim over other people, who must respect it regardless of their wishes. Autonomy allows for an individual's right to self-determination, including their right to determine their medical future. It is necessary to attempt to ensure that a patient really understands the information that has been given to them before it can be considered that informed consent has been obtained. Even if a patient is detained for psychiatric treatment, he or she may be capable of understanding and giving or withholding consent to a surgical procedure. Only if a person is considered mentally incapable of this can the surgeon, together with the patient's psychiatric team, make a decision that they consider to be in the patient's best interests. While the views of children should be considered and treated with respect, it is accepted that, in many cases, they may not be making a properly considered decision. It is for their parents or guardians to consent to or refuse treatment. Only when the surgeon considers that the parents or guardians may not be acting in the child's best interests may this be contested; 16-year-old adolescents are generally deemed capable of giving an informed consent and can sign a document for themselves.

1.18 ACD

Single-blinding refers to the patient not knowing which treatment he/she is receiving. Double-blinding is said to occur when both the patient and the investigator are unaware which treatment the patient is receiving. A trial participant can withdraw at any time. A control group is a group of patients observed after not receiving the index treatment. Historical controls are not as reliable as a group randomised to control.

2 AUDIOLOGY

2.1 CD
Acoustic neuromas arise from Schwann cells, most commonly from the superior vestibular nerve. The sex incidence is equal, and the peak age incidence is between 40 and 60. The most common otological symptom is progressive unilateral deafness, with vertigo being rare; 60% have been shown to be static on regular MRI scanning.

Hitselberger's sign (hypoaesthesia of the posterior canal wall) should raise the suspicion of acoustic neuroma.

2.2 B
Caloric testing is side-specific testing of the semicircular canals, via infusion of water at different temperatures into each external auditory canal. It produces its effects by movement of the endolymph, although what causes this movement is still under debate. The patient is positioned at 30° to the horizontal, and water at 30 °C and 44 °C is infused into opposite canals, separately, for 40 seconds. The resulting nystagmus is timed in each case. The expected response with cold water is nystagmus with the fast phase to the opposite side, while with hot water it is nystagmus with the fast phase to the same side (cold – opposite; warm – same, or COWS). A reduced or absent response indicates pathology in the side being infused.

2.3 CDE
In clinical testing of hearing, the non-tested ear should always be masked if possible. Tuning fork tests should be conducted at 512 Hz; lateral localisation in Weber's test indicates either a conductive loss of > 10 dB in that ear, or a sensorineural loss in the opposite ear. Rinne's test is negative if there is a conductive loss of > 20 dB, but it may also be negative if there is a severe sensorineural loss (false negative – owing to contralateral bone conduction); masking will convert a false-negative Rinne's test into a positive one. Stenger's test involves the simultaneous presentation of two identical tones to both ears at different intensities – because the ear only hears the louder one, a subject with feigned hearing loss will report hearing nothing, whereas someone with true unilateral hearing loss will report hearing the tone in the good ear.

2.4 A
Evoked response audiometry comprises three main techniques. Electrocochleography involves placing a needle through the eardrum and the measurement of the resultant potential. It is used to accurately determine thresholds and to investigate Ménière's disease, where an increase in the summating potential is seen. Brainstem electrical response audiometry measures brain signals produced to sound stimuli, and can be used to exclude acoustic neuroma – however, MRI scanning is more sensitive and specific. Cortical evoked response audiometry also involves the measurement of brain responses, this time in the cortex. None of the tests requires a general anaesthetic; in fact the cortical response is impossible with it.

2.5 D

Over 80% of octogenarians would benefit from hearing aids but only a quarter possesses them. Improvements such as digital hearing aids and the new internal vibrating sound bridge will improve hearing in the future, but so far they are not widely available. Bone conduction aids do not vibrate the skull directly – this requires an osseo-integrated, or bone-anchored aid. It is preferable to provide bilateral hearing aids for bilateral loss, but cost precludes this in the NHS.

2.6 CE

Impedance audiometry involves varying the pressure in the external canal, while drum compliance is measured by the amount of sound energy reflected. Maximum compliance occurs at minimum pressure difference across the eardrum. The resultant curve may peak around 0 mm H_2O (type A), may be flat (type B, suggesting glue ear or perforation) or may peak at a negative pressure (type C, indicating eustachian tube dysfunction). The stapedial reflex is also tested – its presence indicates an intact brainstem and facial nerve. Lastly, static compliance is performed – this measures the difference between the maximum compliance, and the compliance at 200 mm H_2O – a figure > 2 ml indicates perforation.

2.7 AB

Stenger's test involves the simultaneous presentation of two identical tones to both good and 'bad' ears – a report of hearing no sound indicates a non-organic loss. There is usually at least 20 dB between the reflex threshold and the pure tone threshold – less indicates a non-organic loss.

2.8 C

Otoacoustic emissions arise from the outer hair cells, and represent the ear's active response to sounds and their processing. There are numerous classes of OAE, but distortion product OAEs give quick information about specific frequencies, whereas transient evoked OAEs are useful for screening.

2.9 None

An age-related reduction in the amount of inner and outer hair cells results in a loss of hearing, which is worse for high frequencies. Around 20% of those in their eighth decade are affected, but only 20% of those who require them actually use hearing aids.

2.10 BCD

Pure tone audiometry is conducted by decreasing a particular frequency pip in 10-dB intervals until no tone is heard. The tone is then increased in 5-dB intervals until half of the pips are heard. Results are usually given in the dB HL scale, which adjusts for the expected level of hearing so that 0 dB is normal at any given frequency – so a flat curve is a normal result. The dB SPL curve is not flat in normal individuals, as the ear detects sound better in the middle frequencies. Masking is best performed at frequencies close to those being tested.

The Carhart effect is the additional bone conduction given by an intact ossicular chain, leading to an apparent improvement in bone conduction after reconstruction of the ossicular chain.

2.11 B

Sudden hearing loss may be conductive, sensorineural or mixed, and usually only one ear is affected; 60% recover spontaneously. If both ears are affected, this is a medical emergency and the patient should be admitted to hospital. Early empirical treatment with steroids, vasodilators and antibiotics is often given, although there is no specific evidence for its effectiveness.

2.12 ABCD

Up to a third of people are affected at some time by tinnitus. Usually the pitch of tinnitus is found to be around the frequency of any hearing loss. A hearing aid may help, with maximum gain at the frequency of the hearing loss. Hyperacusis is present in 40% of patients with tinnitus.

2.13 D

Vertigo is the hallucination of movement. The semicircular canals contain cilia, and the utricle and saccule also contain otoconia to detect linear acceleration. Most of balance information is due to visual input, and this, along with the vestibular and proprioceptive input, is co-ordinated by the brain.

Hallpike's manoeuvre is used to diagnose benign positional vertigo, and caloric testing is used to test vestibular function.

2.14 ACDE

The most common causes of conductive deafness include wax, acute otitis media, secretory otitis media, chronic otitis media, barotrauma, otosclerosis and injuries to the tympanic membrane and otitis externa. Less common causes include tumours of the middle ear and traumatic ossicular dislocation. Sensorineural deafness is caused by a number of things, including infections such as mumps, herpes zoster, meningitis and syphilis. Other causes of sensorineural deafness include congenital (maternal rubella), cytomegalovirus, toxoplasmosis, prolonged exposure to loud noises, drugs (aspirin, aminoglycosides), Ménière's disease, head injury and acoustic neuroma. Metabolic causes of sensorineural deafness include diabetes and hypothyroidism. In Paget's disease there may be a mixed hearing loss, ie conduction and sensorineural deafness. This may be due to ankylosis of the stapes, or compression of cranial nerve VIII in the auditory foramen by bone.

3 OTOLOGY

3.1 BCDE

Cholesteatoma may be congenital or acquired. It is keratinising squamous epithelia in the middle ear, with the potential to absorb and replace normal middle ear tissue. It may erode through the round window into the labyrinth, resulting in a positive fistula test. Conductive deafness may result from erosion of the middle ear structures, and sensory deafness may result from the migration of toxins into the inner ear.

Treatment is usually complete surgical excision via some form of mastoidectomy, although for mild disease suction clearance may completely cure the patient.

3.2 BE

Streptococcus pneumoniae is the most common cause of ASOM (40% of cases) with *Haemophilus influenzae* causing 30%. Infants have a short, wide eustachian tube, making them more at risk, and teething is also a risk factor. So the peak incidence is between 3 and 7 years. Treatment is with antibiotics; decongestants have a theoretical role which has not been proved.

Gradenigo's syndrome is a rare complication of ASOM, resulting from petrositis of the petrous apex of the temporal bone. The ipsilateral abducent nerve and trigeminal nerve lie nearby, and involvement causes paralysis of the external rectus muscle, and pain in the trigeminal nerve area.

3.3 D

Complications of CSOM may be extracranial (eg tympanosclerosis, facial nerve palsy or labyrinthitis) or intracranial (eg lateral sinus thrombosis, meningitis or abscess). Infection may spread through the oval or round windows, around the arteries, or via the bone. A facial palsy may result from the compression of a dehiscent facial nerve. There is a 1:3500 risk of intracranial abscess with CSOM. A CT scan will show mastoid disease and an MRI scan will show the extent of a lateral sinus thrombosis and an intracranial abscess.

Treatment of suspected complications usually involves antibiotic therapy in the first instance – with no response, surgery may be necessary.

3.4 ADE

A labyrinthine fistula is a bony erosion of the labyrinthine capsule to expose, but not breach, the endosteum of the labyrinth. The Tullio phenomenon is the experience of vertigo in response to loud sounds. A positive fistula sign is shown by the patient deviating eyes away from the side being tested, caused by pressure transmission via labyrinthine fluid. Labyrinthitis causes the patient to look towards the affected side, as this lessens the corrective drive and hence the nystagmus. If a cerebral abscess is suspected, a CT or MRI scan may be indicated.

3.5 ACD

Mastoidectomy is an operation on the mastoid air cells to remove disease. Either an en-aural or postaural incision is used. The cortical mastoidectomy is used for the treatment of acute mastoiditis without cholesteatoma. The modified radical mastoidectomy is used for the treatment of cholesteatoma, and the combined-approach tympanoplasty involves the extension of a cortical mastoidectomy via a posterior tympanotomy. A mastoidectomy with posterior tympanotomy is also required to insert a cochlear implant. Some hearing may be preserved by putting the drum in contact with head of the stapes (a type III tympanoplasty) or by reconstructing the ossicular chain.

3.6 BE

The aetiology of Ménière's disease is still not fully understood, but there appears to be an expansion of the endolymphatic compartment of the inner ear. This leads to temporary damage to the hair cells, and low frequencies are lost first. Classically there is episodic vertigo, tinnitus and hearing loss, along with a sensation of fullness in the ear. It most commonly presents in the fifth decade. The glycerol dehydration test dehydrates the cochlea, and improvement of symptoms is further evidence for Ménière's.

3.7 AD

Many medical treatments of Ménière's disease have not been conclusively proved to work. However, there is evidence to support the control of salt intake. Surgical treatments are equally open to question, and endolymphatic sac surgery may only work by placebo effect. In contrast, gentamicin application to destroy the vestibular labyrinth does have some effect on the disease.

3.8 BCDFG

The sensory nerve supply of the ear is complex – the lower half of the pinna is supplied by the greater auricular nerve (C2, C3), and the upper half from the lesser occipital nerve medially and the auriculotemporal nerve laterally (from the mandibular nerve). The external auditory meatus is supplied by the auriculotemporal nerve and branches of the facial nerve and the vagus nerve (Alderman's nerve). The medial tympanic membrane is supplied by Jacobson's nerve (via the glossopharyngeal nerves and the tympanic plexus) and by the facial nerve. Dental disease irritating the trigeminal nerve is the most common referred cause of otalgia.

3.9 BDE

The external auditory meatus has ceruminous glands in the outer third of the ear, and contains *Staphylococcus albus* as a commensal. Its pH is normally between 3 and 5. Aluminium acetate drops may be used to treat *Pseudomonas* infection, and they work by lowering the pH. Mastoiditis characteristically causes downward and forward displacement of the pinna, although this may be difficult to discern.

Malignant otitis externa is a spreading infection involving osteomyelitis of the skull base. It is common in diabetics and usually caused by *Pseudomonas aeruginosa*. It is treated by iv antibiotics.

3.10 None

Otitis media has its highest prevalence at age 2, decreasing with age, although the peak age of presentation is 3–6 years. It is caused by a reduction in pressure in the middle ear, leading to an inflammatory response in the mucosa and the production of thick mucus ('glue'); 90% of cases resolve spontaneously, although there may be multiple relapses before this happens. Grommets may be used to treat otitis media – swimming does not increase the risk of infection, but soapy water may do. Multiple grommet insertions and bleeding is associated with tympanosclerosis.

3.11 BC

Around 80% of temporal bone fractures involve a longitudinal component, usually from a lateral skull blow. Facial nerve injuries are uncommon but CSF otorrhoea may be present. Transverse fractures arise most commonly from blows to the front or back of the skull, and commonly lead to more serious nerve injuries such as facial nerve palsies or deafness. Temporal bone fractures often cause facial nerve weakness but this is not an indication for immediate exploration.

3.12 CE

Otosclerosis is an autosomal dominant condition affecting bone derived from the otic capsule; there is a 2:1 female:male ratio. It leads to clinical symptoms in 0.5–2% of the population, although 10% have at least subclinical disease; 10% of cases display Schwartze's sign, a pink tinge to the tympanic membrane from dilated blood vessels; 85% of patients have bilateral disease. Taste is not affected, but may be damaged in the subsequent stapedectomy.

3.13 ABD

Aminoglycosides may be predominantly cochleotoxic (neomycin) or vestibulotoxic (gentamicin). The relative balance of each depends on the number of anime and methylamine groups respectively. Susceptibility is transmitted by women through mitochondria. Ears may be protected by antioxidant prophylaxis.

Loop diuretics can cause ototoxicity in high doses, although the high-tone hearing loss is usually reversible.

3.14 AD

A perilymph fistula is a leak into the middle ear arising from the oval (most commonly) or round window. It leads to a progressive sensorineural hearing loss, and may be treated by plugging with a graft after tympanotomy. It may be associated with a congenital deformity, for example Mondini's dysplasia.

3.15 ABD

Tympanoplasty aims to eradicate middle ear disease and to reconstruct the hearing mechanism by means of autografting or prosthesis placement. Homografting has been used in the past, but is now contraindicated because of the theoretical risk of Creutzfeldt–Jakob disease. Diving is contraindicated after reconstruction, as the repair may be displaced.

3.16 AF
The axons supplying taste over the anterior two-thirds of the tongue and secretomotor fibres to the submandibular and sublingual salivary glands (the parotid is innervated by cranial nerve IX) are found in the chorda tympani nerve. The chorda tympani courses across the tympanic membrane beneath the mucous membrane of the middle ear after leaving the facial canal approximately 0.5 cm above the stylomastoid foramen. It exits the middle ear by passing through the petrotympanic fissure medially, and runs forwards on the medial side of the spine of the sphenoid bone. After entering the infratemporal fossa, it merges with the lingual nerve. The chorda tympani, therefore, is not related to the parotid gland. It also escapes injury when the facial nerve is compressed within the most distal part of the facial canal (the facial canal is the passageway of the facial nerve after it emerges from the internal auditory meatus).

3.17 B
Earache from acute tonsillitis is due to referred pain along the glossopharyngeal nerve, which runs in the tonsillar bed and which sends a tympanic branch to the tympanic plexus in the middle ear. The other nerves are not involved.

3.18 A
Acute otitis media is very common, especially in children, in whom presentation may be in the form of generalised malaise, pyrexia or gastrointestinal upset. Otalgia and hearing loss are more common features in adults. The causative organisms are usually *Streptococcus pneumoniae* or *S. haemophilus*. The first-line treatment is a broad-spectrum antibiotic, eg amoxicillin. Myringotomy is only advocated once perforation has occurred. If the acute phase does not settle, a more chronic infection develops and, in rare instances, a cholesteatoma may form.

3.19 All true
Middle ear infection is one of the commonest causes of a brain abscess (temporal, cerebellar). This may subsequently give rise to the clinical features of raised intracranial pressure, cranial neuropathies (III–VII) and visual disturbance. Sudden deafness may be caused by a middle ear effusion.

3.20 BCD
The medial wall, which separates the middle from the internal ear, contains the oval window and promontory. The promontory is the rounded projection of the first turn of the cochlea. Also medially, the internal auditory meatus carries the facial nerve. The floor is a thin bone separating the middle ear form the bulb of the jugular vein. Anteriorly, a thin bone wall separates the cavity from the internal carotid artery.

4 RHINOLOGY

4.1 BE

Allergic rhinitis affects the mucous membranes of the nose. It is a typical type I hypersensitivity reaction, affecting 30% of the western population. The Fc portion of the IgE molecule joins to mast cells and basophils, while the Fab portion combines with the allergen, triggering a chain of events leading to the release of arachidonic acid metabolites. This produces congestion, oedema and rhinorrhoea. There may be polyps but these are more usually associated with intrinsic rhinitis.

Treatment is medical in the first instance – oral antihistamines and topical steroid spray may have an effect, as may other mast cell stabilisers and anticholinergics. Oral steroids should be used only for short-term treatment. Turbinate surgery may offer some relief in unresponsive cases.

4.2 BCDE

This common ENT problem is usually of idiopathic origin. The upper parts of the nose are supplied by the internal carotid artery via the ethmoidal arteries, and the rest of the nasal mucosa is supplied by the external carotid via the greater palatine, sphenopalatine and superior labial arteries. A rare cause is HHT – epistaxis is common, and treatment may require oestrogens or mucosal skin grafts.

Treatment of epistaxis is initially conservative, with external pressure or anterior or posterior packing to stem the flow. Posterior packing raises the risk of eustachian tube infection, and antibiotic cover should be given. Further bleeding despite packing necessitates surgical intervention, eg endoscopic sphenopalatine artery ligation, anterior ethmoidal artery clipping via a medial orbital incision, or even external carotid artery ligation via the neck.

4.3 BCE

Wegener's granulomatosis is a necrotising vasculitis involving lesions of the respiratory tracts and glomerulonephritis. c-ANCA is a relatively sensitive test (91%) for the disease. Three-system involvement and biopsy of an active area of disease is necessary for diagnosis. It is thought to have a viral precipitant.

Sarcoidosis shows non-caseating granulomas on biopsy, and the Kveim test is usually positive.

4.4 AC

Any form of rhinitis may initiate the formation of nasal polyps, which are folds of insensitive swollen mucosa. There may be a link with immune function, and polyps are commonly associated with asthma and aspirin sensitivity. In a child they may be signs of cystic fibrosis. Treatment is with intranasal steroids or short courses of oral steroids in the first instance – surgery in the form of polypectomy may be necessary later. Antochoanal polyps are usually solitary, and emerge from the lining of the maxillary sinus.

4.5 ABCD

The nasal bone is the most commonly fractured bone in the body. Assault is the most frequent cause. Most are treated by manipulation between 1–2 weeks after the initial injury, but some may require open reduction. A septal haematoma may be treated by aspiration, but if it repeatedly returns it should be formally incised, drained and sutured. A numbness below the eye is a sign of infraorbital nerve damage, and a blow-out fracture should be excluded. Clear rhinorrhoea is a sign of a CSF leak through the cribriform plate, and some may require surgical repair.

4.6 BCE

FESS eliminates the need for mucosal stripping, leading to a better functional result. Many operations may be performed by this method, including pituitary surgery, sphenopalatine artery ligation and dacrocystorhinostomy. There are still complications, however. A CSF leak, if identified at the time of surgery, should be repaired immediately, using a turbinate flap or graft, or glue. FESS in the nose may be performed front-to-back (Messerklinger technique) or back-to-front (Wigand technique). Postoperative nasal douching to remove crusts is often advised.

4.7 BDE

Septal perforation usually affects the anterior cartilaginous part. If Wegener's granulomatosis is suspected, an ANCA test may be indicated. Trauma from nose-picking is a common cause.

Treatment with surgical closure is difficult, and other methods may be tried – medical treatment, silastic button placement, or enlargement if whistling is the major symptom.

4.8 CDE

Some 50% of sinonasal tumours are squamous cell carcinomas. Working with hardwood is a risk factor for developing ethmoidal adenocarcinoma. Most tumours arise from the upper jaw. The most important benign tumour is the inverted papilloma, comprising a papilliferous mass with deep invaginations into the stroma. These may be treated with endoscopic resection, although formerly they were treated by lateral rhinostomy. Sinonasal tumours present late owing to their location and rarity.

4.9 ACE

The usual causative organisms of acute sinusitis are *Streptococcus pneumoniae* and *Haemophilus influenzae*. Treatment is often with broad-spectrum antibiotics in the first instance.

In chronic cases, removal of the mucosa may be indicated, although endoscopic surgery can provide a less invasive solution. Thickened mucosa is a meaningless finding in itself, and CT scans should not be used to diagnose sinusitis.

Kartagener's syndrome is a risk factor for sinusitis, because of cilial dysfunction and consequent inadequate sinus drainage.

4.10 BDE

Olfaction is provided by the roof of the nasal cavity, which is supplied by the olfactory nerves. Gustation is served by the taste buds, and the glossopharyngeal and facial nerves – the front of the tongue detects sweet and salt tastes; the posterior detects bitter tastes; and the lateral tongue detects sour tastes. Common chemical sensation is served by branches of the trigeminal nerve, and tends to react to unpleasant stimuli.

4.11 BCDEFG

Maxillary sinus carcinoma tends to affect African, Japanese and Arabic populations. It is much rarer in Western Europe and the USA. Ninety per cent of cancers of the sinus affect the maxillary and ethmoid sinuses, with only 10% affecting the frontal and sphenoid sinuses. Definite aetiological factors include hardwood dust and nickel. Other implicated factors include radiation, mustard gas production and materials used in bootmaking. The clinical features include: nasal obstruction; epistaxis; toothache; loosening of the teeth; destruction of bone, which may lead to proptosis, enophthalmos or diplopia; invasion of the nerves causing numbness of the facial palate; and invasion of the infratemporal fossa causing trismus. In 10% of cases there is metastatic involvement of the lymph nodes.

4.12 CD

Epistaxis results from a wide range of local and systemic conditions. It may be a presenting feature of haematological disease, eg leukaemia or lymphoma. The most common site of epistaxis is the anterior nasal area (Little's area). If bleeding does not stop with pressure, then packing (anteronasal or posteronasal) is required. A Foley urinary catheter, not a Fogarty catheter, is useful for staunching the haemorrhage. Sedation should be avoided as this may compromise respiration.

4.13 BDF

The nasopharynx lies behind the nasal cavity above the soft palate. The nasopharynx contains the pharyngeal tonsil (adenoid), salpingopharyngeal fold (produced by the salpingopharyngeus muscle), and the pharyngeal recess posterior to the tubal elevation and adjacent to the internal carotid artery. The pyramidal fossae lie in the laryngopharynx. The pharyngeal branch of the cranial nerve VII, coming from the pterygopalatine ganglion, supplies the mucosa of the nasopharynx.

4.14 BCE

Olfactory neuroblastoma is a rare tumour of the olfactory neural crest cells, and usually presents with unilateral nasal obstruction and sinusitis symptoms, along with some degree of anosmia. All ages are affected. It almost always involves the cribriform plate, and so resection will usually involve a craniofacial approach.

5 LARYNGOLOGY

5.1 ABDE

Thyroglossal cysts lie along the track of the obliterated thyroglossal tract, and most lie in the midline – however, 9% lie on the left and 1% on the right. They may contain elements of thyroid tissue. A technetium or radio-iodine scan may therefore confirm the diagnosis, although an ultrasound scan may also be used. Clinically, they move with both swallowing and tongue protrusion, as they are attached to the thyroglossal tract remnant and the larynx – however, a dermoid cyst attached to the hyoid may be misdiagnosed as a thyroglossal cyst.

The operation of choice is Sistrunk's operation, which involves excision of the whole of the tract together with the median third of the hyoid bone. If this is done, the recurrence rate should be < 10%.

5.2 ACD

There are many theories regarding the origin of branchial cysts, but the most popular one at present suggests that islands of squamous epithelium within lymph nodes cause their formation. They usually present in young adults, with 60% on the left side and 60% in men. They lie deep to the anterior border of the sternocleidomastoid muscle, at the junction of the upper third and middle two-thirds. Infection occurs in a quarter of cases, and excision is indicated when inflammation has settled.

5.3 ABD

Chemodectomas arise from nerve tissue on the medial side of the carotid bulb (carotid body tumours), from the vagus nerve (glomus vagale tumours) or the ganglion nodosum just below the jugular foramen (glomus jugulare tumours). Carotid body tumours are more common at high altitude, for example in Bolivia. They are almost always benign, although mass effects may lead to pressure on skull base structures. An arteriogram is the first-line investigation, and it often shows a splayed carotid bifurcation.

If necessary, it may be possible to resect the tumour, with graft replacement of the involved carotid artery portion if required.

5.4 BC

Neck nodes are divided into various levels, and their enlargement from neoplasia can be classified by the UICC system as follows:

N0   regional nodes not palpable
N1   movable single ipsilateral or bilateral nodes < 3 cm
N2   movable ipsilateral or bilateral nodes
a   single ipsilateral node 3–6 cm diameter
b   multiple ipsilateral nodes < 6 cm diameter
c   bilateral or contralateral nodes < 6 cm diameter
N3   nodes > 6 cm diameter

After a careful search, up to 10% of patients have no identifiable primary source. Treatment will depend to some extent on the primary, but N1 nodes may be treated by radiotherapy alone, although some prefer a modified radical neck dissection. N2 is an indication for a neck dissection, and N3 may indicate the need for a palliative procedure.

5.5 BC

ENT cosmetic surgery operations include rhinoplasty, pinnaplasty, facial reanimation and facelifts (rhytidectomy). Pinnaplasty is not carried out before the age of 3 years, and usually before school age. The most important part of the treatment is the postoperative head dressing, which must be tight and must remain in place for 7–14 days. Facial reanimation is carried out for intractable facial palsy and involves a combination of facial nerve grafting, suspension of the angle of the mouth by transposition of temporalis muscle of tissue patch, and eyelid procedures. At least a year should be given to make sure that no improvement will occur. The modern rhytidectomy involves elevating the SMAS to give a more natural and tension-free result.

5.6 AC

Facial nerve palsy is usually due to Bell's palsy (55%), although this is a diagnosis of exclusion. Treatment usually involves a short course of high-dose steroids, with artificial tears to lubricate the eye, and aciclovir if a viral aetiology cannot be excluded. Neoplasia may be a cause (6%), arising from within or outside the nerve. 'Crocodile tears' or masticatory lacrimation has no bearing on the prognosis; electromyogram response in the early stages is the only reliable indicator of recovery. Grading is carried out using the House–Brackmann classification. If there is no response to medical treatment, a facial reanimation procedure may be necessary.

5.7 CD

Ninety per cent of hypopharyngeal tumours are squamous cell carcinomas. A strong association with tobacco and alcohol has not yet been proved, in contrast to other upper tract tumours. There is, however, an association with PVPK syndrome, in that 2% of patients with the disease will suffer postcricoid carcinoma. Staging is similar to other carcinomas, in that a tumour > 4 cm diameter is classified as T3.

Watchful waiting is not an option with hypopharyngeal tumours – patients will always require some treatment to the neck if a cure is to be achieved. Surgical resection usually involves some permanent derangement of thyroid or parathyroid hormones, and patients often require lifelong supplementation.

5.8 AD

The most common feature of laryngeal carcinoma is hoarseness, although dyspnoea and stridor may eventually also be present. Staging usually requires direct visualisation of the tumour via panendoscopy – a fixed vocal cord in supraglottic or glottic tumours indicates a T3 lesion. Glottis tumours rarely metastasise until they have spread superiorly or inferiorly, as the glottis has only limited lymph drainage. Smaller lesions may be treated by radiotherapy alone, but larger ones often require a neck dissection combined with a total laryngectomy, which includes removal of the thyroid gland.

5.9 ABE

Nasopharyngeal carcinoma usually arises from the fossa of Rosenmuller. Highest incidence is in the Southern Chinese people, with the Epstein–Barr virus and salted preserved fish being implicated as causal agents. Radiotherapy is the treatment of choice, although a radical neck dissection may occasionally be necessary.

Angiofibroma is a benign tumour made up of vascular tissue and arising from the back of the nose. It affects young men, and always involves the sphenopalatine foramen; indeed this may be the site of origin.

5.10 C

A radical neck dissection refers to the removal of lymph nodes in the anterior and posterior triangles, along with the submandibular gland, the spinal accessory nerve, and internal jugular vein and the sternocleidomastoid muscle. To omit at least one of these removals makes it a modified radical neck dissection. Intracranial pressure rises threefold in a unilateral dissection, and rises tenfold in a bilateral one – so bilateral dissections are not undertaken unless they are completely necessary. Frozen shoulder is a late complication, although removal of the spinal accessory nerve results in an immediate loss of shoulder shrugging.

5.11 DF

The parapharyngeal space extends from the skull base to the diaphragm, and is divided by the styloid process into posterior and anterior portions – the posterior part contains the carotid sheath. The infratemporal fossa is bounded superiorly by the greater wing of the sphenoid. Prevertebral abscesses are caused by TB; retropharyngeal and parapharyngeal abscesses are most commonly caused by tonsillitis and upper respiratory tract infections, and submandibular abscesses (Ludwig's angina) are most commonly caused by dental infections.

5.12 BE

Most malignant tumours of the oral cavity are squamous cell carcinomas. Alcohol consumption and smoking are risk factors. The commonest sites are the lateral border of the tongue and the floor of the mouth. In almost all cases of oral carcinoma, treatment should be given to the neck nodes on the form of radiotherapy or a node dissection. Treatment to both sides of the neck may be necessary, given the extensive crossover of lymph drainage from the oral cavity area.

5.13 None

The oropharynx is bordered by the posterior third of the tongue and the valleculae anteriorly, the anterior and posterior tonsillar pillars laterally, and the hard palate and aryepiglottic folds posteriorly. Most carcinoma is diagnosed as squamous cell carcinoma (85%) with 10% being NHL. Investigations indicated are MRI, FNA cytology, and panendoscopy.

5.14 BCD

Indications for tracheostomy are airway obstruction, protection of the tracheobronchial tree, and decreasing ventilatory insufficiency. There are many different types of tube, and some are fenestrated for vocalisation. Paediatric tubes are usually non-cuffed. The first change of the tube should occur at 48 hours.

Percutaneous tracheostomy is associated with lower overall costs than standard tracheostomy.

5.15 BCD

Adductor palsy may be treated with medialisation – if it is on both sides it may lead to aspiration. The recurrent laryngeal nerve supplies sensation below the cords and most intrinsic laryngeal muscles – the superior laryngeal nerve supplies sensation above the cords and the cricothyroid muscle.

5.16 BC

Respiratory papillomatosis is the most common benign tumour of the larynx, and usually occurs initially between the ages of 0 and 5 years. It tends to regress with age. Treatment with laser surgery may be necessary. Papillomas in adults are subject to malignant transformation, especially if the patient smokes.

5.17 CE
Pharyngeal pouches arise from a posterior herniation of pharyngeal mucosa through a defect between thyropharyngeus and cricopharyngeus (Killian's dehiscence) in the inferior constrictor. They are best diagnosed by a barium swallow, and may be treated in a number of ways, including endoscopic division. A cricopharyngeal myotomy may be performed to prevent reformation of the pouch.

5.18 B
Primary Sjögren's syndrome means the existence of symptoms (xerostomia, xerophthalmia) without an underlying connective tissue disorder – 'secondary' implies the presence of a disorder.

Papillary cystadenoma is a benign disease of the parotid gland (Warthin's tumour).

Incisional biopsies should not be performed as there is a risk of spreading the tumour; a fine-needle biopsy is often useful.

5.19 ABC
Eighty per cent of all salivary gland tumours originate in the parotid and, of these, 80% are benign. The peak incidence of pleomorphic adenoma is in the fifth decade. In the minor salivary glands only 50% are benign; 10% are bilateral in the case of Warthin's tumours. Mucoepidermoid carcinoma is the most common malignant parotid tumour, followed by adenoid cystic carcinoma.

5.20 ACFG
OSA is defined as > 30 apnoeic episodes in 7 hours, or if the apnoea index is > 5 (number of periods of apnoea per hour). It may be caused by peripheral airway obstruction or central respiratory depression, and the two must be differentiated if effective treatment is to be given. OSA affects 6% of men, while snoring affects 60% of men over 60. Müller's manoeuvre is vigorous inhalation against a closed mouth and nose, with a flexible scope used to observe the movement of the hypopharynx.

If CPAP is needed, it is important not to carry out uvulopalatopharyngoplasty, as this then prevents effective application of CPAP. Severe OSA may require tracheostomy, although this is rare.

5.21 BCD
Graves' disease is an IgG-mediated reaction against TSH receptors. Hashimoto's thyroiditis causes hypothyroidism and gives a firm uniform enlargement. Thyroid surgery puts the external superior laryngeal nerve and the recurrent laryngeal nerve at risk. Radionucleotide scanning shows uptake of I^{123} and can differentiate between a 'cold' nodule (more likely to be malignant) and a 'hot' one.

Prendred's syndrome is the association of congenital hypothyroidism with high-tone deafness.

5.22 D
Papillary carcinoma is the most common thyroid malignancy, and typically spreads via the lymph system. It may be adequately treated by a subtotal thyroidectomy in the case of a T1 lesion. Follicular carcinoma spreads via the bloodstream, but cannot be definitively diagnosed on FNA, owing to the confusion with adenoma – a lobectomy is therefore usually required.

Medullary carcinoma is associated with MEN type 2.

5.23 A
Tracheal stenosis following tracheostomy may occur at three possible sites – the level of the stoma, the level of the cuff and at the tip of the tube. The incidence is approximately 10%. The standard approach is a 2-cm transverse incision 2 cm above the sternal notch. The thyroid isthmus may need to be tied as it lies over the second and third tracheal rings. This has no effect on the thyroid status of the patient. In adults the tracheostomy is placed between the second and fourth tracheal rings, and in children at the second and third tracheal rings. The cough reflex is lost in someone with a tracheostomy and the patient is unable to clear secretions from the tracheobronchial tree – frequent suction is therefore necessary.

5.24 B
Emergency tracheostomy is a formal operation and should be carried out under controlled circumstances under general anaesthetic. However, percutaneous tracheostomy is performed under local anaesthetic in some centres. It is useful in enabling adequate toilet of the lungs, and reduction in dead space may aid weaning from ventilation. Anatomical dead space of the respiratory tract refers to all areas not involved in gas exchange, eg the oropharynx.

5.25 CDEF
Papillary carcinoma accounts for 70% of all thyroid tumours. It usually presents in children and young adults. Medullary carcinoma of the thyroid is associated with multiple endocrine neoplasia (MEN 2A and 2B). Following unilateral lobectomy or total thyroidec-tomy, papillary carcinomas are treated with thyroxine to suppress TSH levels, thereby reducing recurrence. Most patients with thyroid tumour are euthyroid and, although hyper-thyroidism can occur, it is relatively uncommon. The combination of adequate sampling with an experienced cytopathologist makes FNA a useful first-line modality for the detection of tumour cells. Surgical resection is the mainstay of therapy for papillary carcinoma of the thyroid. Radioactive iodine may be used as an adjuvant or to treat metastases. Because thyroglobulin is only synthesised by thyroid tissue, it has been proved to be a useful tumour marker. Tall and Hürthle cells are aggressive variants of papillary thyroid cancer. They have a greater potential for malignant behaviour.

5.26 ACDE

The submandibular gland is a lobulated gland made up of a superficial and a deep part, which are continuous with each other around the posterior border of the mylohyoid muscle. The gland is partly infralateral, enclosed in an investing layer of deep cervical fascia, platysma muscle and skin. Laterally it is crossed by the cervical branch of the facial nerve and vein. The facial artery is related to the posterior and superior aspects of the superficial part of the gland.

5.27 BC

Bilateral vocal cord paralysis is a recognised complication of thyroidectomy, and is caused by damage to the recurrent laryngeal nerves. In a partial unilateral paralysis of the recurrent laryngeal nerve, the cords lie in the midline. A complete recurrent laryngeal nerve paralysis would cause the cords to lie midway between the normal resting position and the midline. Patients must therefore be assessed immediately for airway obstruction, which manifests as stridor. In the longer term, laser arytenoidectomy provides the best compromise between a patent airway and a functional voice. Diphtheria may cause upper airway obstruction, but does so by the production of a thick fibrinopurulent film over the lumen.

5.28 ACDE

Sjögren's syndrome manifests as dry eyes and dry mouth. It is associated with many immunological conditions, most commonly rheumatoid arthritis but also SLE. It may occur alone in the absence of rheumatoid arthritis. Rheumatoid factor is usually present, even in primary disease. Anti-Ro antibodies and circulating immune complexes are also found in the blood. The exocrine glands are infiltrated with lymphocytes and plasma cells, thereby causing their destruction and resulting in dry eyes and dry mouth. Frey's syndrome occurs after parotid surgery.

6 PAEDIATRICS

6.1 B

Adenoids consist of lymphoid tissue at the junction of the roof and posterior wall of the nasopharynx. Enlarged adenoids may present with symptoms of nasal obstruction or eustachian tube dysfunction. The classic 'adenoidal facies' is actually rare. A lateral soft tissue X-ray may give an idea of the size of the adenoids, but the only reliable means of assessment is examination under anaesthetic. Indications for removal include nasal obstruction, otitis media, and sleep apnoea; a cleft palate is a contraindication for removal, as, in these children, the adenoids may assist in closure of the nasopharynx from the oropharynx. Complications of adenoidectomy include haemorrhage, eustachian tube stenosis and hypernasal speech.

6.2 ABCE

Choanal atresia is a failure of rupture of the bucconasal membrane before birth. It is usually unilateral, in which case diagnosis may be delayed, but is sometimes bilateral, in which case it presents as an emergency shortly after birth owing to the obligate nasal breathing pattern of the infant. In 50% of cases there is an associated facial palsy, and one-third have laryngotracheal abnormalities. All babies with choanal atresia should be screened for the CHARGE association, namely C – coloboma, H – heart disease, A – choanal atresia, R – retarded growth, G – genital abnormalities, and E – ear abnormalities.

Treatment in symptomatic cases is perforation/drilling of the occlusion, with or without the simultaneous placement of stents. Regular dilation is usually necessary at first, and some centres are using mitomycin-C as an adjuvant treatment to prevent re-stenosis.

6.3 BE

The idea of a 'central' or 'safe' perforation, as opposed to a 'peripheral' or 'unsafe' one, is being superseded by division into mucous/squamous epithelial, and active/inactive disease, and reference to the old terms should be avoided. Grommet insertion is a risk factor for permanent perforation, which occurs in 40% after 2 years, and is associated with an air/bone gap of < 30 dB. Intracranial complications are an equal risk of CSOM, whether or not there is a cholesteatoma associated. CSOM cultures in children reveal that 50% have anaerobic infection, and antibiotics must be used which cover this.

6.4 CD

Cochlear implants comprise an internal implanted array in the inner ear, and an external microphone and transmitter coil. Neural plasticity is the ability of the brain to be programmed to learn tasks, and the ability to listen is lost by the age of 8 years; however, the ability to make speech articulations occurs only if speech is heard by the age of 3 years. So people may be classified as prelingually deaf (deafness occurred before acquiring speech) or postlingually deaf (deafness occurred after acquiring speech). Postlingually deaf individuals may be considered for implantation at any age; however, prelingually deaf individuals should be implanted before the age of 8, or the ability to make sense of auditory stimuli will be lost.

6.5 C

Cystic fibrosis may present as recurrent respiratory tract infection, and chest physiotherapy is an important part of patients' management. Nasal polyps are rarely seen in children and the common cold will produce a bilateral nasal discharge. The most common cause for a unilateral nasal discharge is a foreign body, and if this has been present for some time, it will be associated with a foul smell. The discharge is often bloodstained.

6.6 ABD

Cleft lip has an increasing incidence with 1/750 affected live births. The condition is more common in males. The subsequent risk of future affected children is 5%, rising to 9% with two affected siblings. Cleft lip has an association with palate defects in up to 50% of cases.

6.7 CD

Congenital hearing loss may be sensorineural or conductive, and may be autosomal recessive or dominant, although most are recessive. There are many syndromes recognised, eg Pendred's – an autosomal recessive syndrome where a sensorineural hearing loss is accompanied by a thyroid goitre. The ossicles and pinna form from the first and second branchial arches, and hence hearing disorders may result from abnormalities of these embryological precursors. Intrauterine rubella infection causes a congenital sensorineural hearing loss.

6.8 BE

Epiglottitis is usually caused by *Haemophilus influenzae* type B, despite the advent of the Hib vaccine given at 2 months. The peak incidence is between 3 and 4 years. Clinically, the child will present with a sore throat, leading to muffled voice and respiratory obstruction. The child may be sitting up and dribbling. No attempt should be made to examine the throat, or to distress the child, as laryngospasm may result. The primary concern is to secure a safe airway. Once this is done, iv antibiotics such as chloramphenicol should be started, and the child transferred to intensive care facilities if necessary.

6.9 AD

Ear foreign bodies usually can be removed via suction or hooks, but may occasionally require a postaural incision. Patients with throat foreign bodies should never have a barium swallow because it interferes with future oesophagoscopies, although an Omnopaque swallow may be possible. Oesophageal foreign bodies usually wedge at the cricopharyngeus, but may also occur at the cardia or at the crossing of the left main bronchus. Bronchial foreign bodies usually go down the right main bronchus, as it is larger and straighter.

Lateral neck X-rays show low sensitivity and specificity for foreign bodies, and they should not be used to make management decisions without taking clinical symptoms into account.

6.10 BCD

Stertor is noise originating from the back of the mouth or nose, and may be helped by the insertion of a nasopharyngeal airway. Stridor originates more distally and, if inspiratory, is likely to come from the laryngeal level, with expiratory stridor originating from the tracheal level. Children may suffer from subglottic stenosis, usually owing to trauma, and this may require reconstruction of the airway, perhaps through a laryngotracheal reconstruction. Another cause of stridor is the presence of a vascular ring, which may compress the trachea and oesophagus.

6.11 A

Screening hearing tests are performed at age 7 months (distraction), 2–4 years (distraction/conditioned response) and preschool (pure tone audiometry). Otoacoustic emission testing is suitable for universal screening but has yet not been implemented – it provides an objective hearing test for newborn infants.

Conditioned response audiometry is assessing the response of a child to an auditory stimulus after conditioning – the child of course needs to be awake. Evoked response audiometry is the measurement of brain responses to auditory stimulus, and as such generally needs to be performed with the child under anaesthetic.

6.12 CE

The aetiology of tonsillitis is usually unclear, with many presumed to be due to a viral infection. If the patient is admitted to hospital, a glandular fever test should be performed, and amoxicillin should not be given for fear of precipitating a maculopapular rash. Quinsy is the development of peritonsillar abscess after tonsillitis, and is treated by drainage and antibiotics. Other complications include septicaemia and glomerulonephritis.

6.13 CDE

There is no definite rule, but a child having tonsillitis five times a year for at least 2 years is a good candidate for tonsillectomy. Postoperative haemorrhage occurs in 2% of cases, and is likely to be from the tonsillar branch of the facial artery. Intractable bleeding may require a return to theatre and suturing of the faucial pillars over kaltostat gauze. The voice quality may be affected, because of stiffening of the palate.

6.14 CDE

Children have a larger head, which tends to flex the head on the neck, making airway obstruction more likely. The relatively larger tongue tends to flop back and obstruct the airway in the obtunded child and means there is less room in the mouth when they are being intubated. The larynx is more cephalic (glottis at C3 in infants compared with C6 in adults) and the angle of the jaw is larger in children (140° in infants, 120° in adults), both making intubation more difficult. In addition, the trachea is shorter and the cricoid ring is the narrowest part of the airway (compared with the glottis in the adult).

6.15 AC

Glue ear is a serous viscous effusion that may occur after an episode of acute otitis media. Conditions predisposing to the condition are eustachian tube dysfunction, adenoidal hypertrophy and allergic conditions. Cleft palate has no association.

6.16 ADE

The eustachian tube in a child is shorter and more horizontal. The opening of the auditory tube lies above the soft palate, adjacent to the tubal tonsil. The bony part of the eustachian tube perforates the petrous temporal bone.

6.17 BC

The most likely diagnosis is a thyroglossal cyst. Other differential diagnoses should include epidermal cyst and dermoid cyst. An ultrasound scan is the most useful first-line test. Treatment of thyroglossal cyst is by surgical excision.

6.18 BC

The complication of acute glomerulonephritis following tonsillitis is more common in men. The particular condition has a latency of 1–3 weeks. Group A β-haemolytic streptococcal infection commonly occurs in children > 10 years old. Peritonsillar abscess or quinsy cause medial displacement of the soft palate or uvula. Pulmonary hypertension, heart failure and secondary chronic hypoxia have all been described. Odynophagia and otalgia can also occur. Cholesteatoma is keratinised stratified squamous epithelium growing in the middle ear (which is usually lined by columnar epithelium). It should be treated aggressively as it can be invasive and fatal.

ENT Examination

CONTENTS

ENT Examination

The DO-HNS examination requires candidates to be fluent in basic ENT examination skills. This usually involves an approach starting with introduction to the patient and enquiring whether any areas of interest are tender at all. The examination proceeds with inspection of all relevant areas. Palpation may be necessary, particularly of the neck, but percussion and auscultation are only useful in thyroid examination. You may find it best to state what you are doing for both the patient's and the examiner's benefit as you go along – indeed, the examiner may ask you to do so. This section gives guidelines for examination of the ear, nose, throat and neck.

SECTION 3

Examination of the Ear

1   Introduce yourself to the patient and ask whether the ear is tender anywhere.
2   Inspect the pinna from the side, looking for discharge, swelling, erythema, deformity and endauricular scars. Inspect from the front, comparing it with the other side for symmetry.
3   Move the pinna forwards gently so that the area behind is exposed – look for post-auricular scars and mastoid swelling. Palpate the mastoid process for tenderness.
4   Gently pull the ear superiorly, laterally and posteriorly (in children inferiorly and posteriorly) to straighten the external canal. Use the hand opposite to the side you are examining (ie for the left ear use the right hand). Insert an appropriately sized otoscope with speculum into the outer cartilaginous part of the canal only.
5   Hold the otoscope with its axis pointing upwards and forwards (at 45° to the horizontal) in the same hand as the side you are examining (ie for the left ear hold in the left hand) between the thumb and forefinger (Fig. 1). Brace the little finger of this hand against the side of the patient's head – this gives both you and the patient some security should the head move.
6   Inspect all areas of the external canal and the tympanic membrane. Systematically inspect the handle of the malleus and all four quadrants of the membrane, looking for evidence of perforation, glue ear, tympanosclerosis, cholesteatoma, previous mastoid surgery and grommet in situ. If there is a perforation, note what is visible behind it. If the mastoid cavity can be seen, note whether it is healthy and look for the presence of a facial ridge (ridge behind which lies the facial nerve). You should be able to draw what you see immediately after examining the membrane, and indeed the examiner may ask you to do this.
7   Perform a fistula test by applying reasonably firm pressure over the tragus for a few seconds. Watch for deviation of the eyes away from the examined side and then nystagmus in the direction of the diseased side. This will show if there is a communication between the outer and inner ear. This test can also be done using a pneumatic otoscope (an otoscope with a squeezable rubber air reservoir).
8   Hearing tests should be done, starting with free speech as a distance of 60 cm from the ear (Fig. 2). This should be done by saying bisyllabic words or two-figure numbers in a whispered voice, a normal voice and a loud voice. The patient should repeat what is said, and the test should be stopped when more than 50% of words are repeated correctly. The contralateral ear should be masked with either a Barany noise box or tragal pressure, and the patient should not be able to lip-read the tester.
9   Tuning fork tests are performed with a 256- or a 512-Hz tuning fork struck on the elbow or knee (of the tester). Rinne's test (Fig. 3) compares air with bone conduction – air conduction is assessed with the prongs of the tuning fork in line with, and 2 cm away

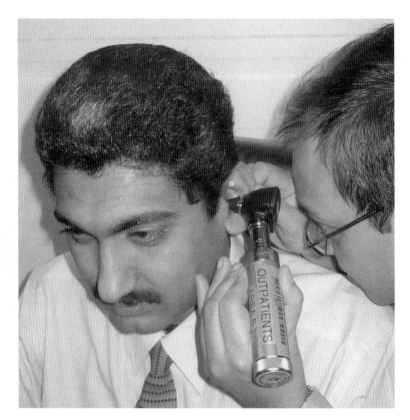

Fig. 1 Otoscopic ear examination

from, the axis of the ear canal. Bone conduction is assessed with the base of the tuning fork pressed against the mastoid process and with pressure applied with the other hand on the contralateral part of the skull. The quickest way is to ask the patient to compare the loudness of air and bone conduction. With normal hearing the air conduction is louder (Rinne-positive), which also occurs when there is sensorineural loss on that side. A negative Rinne response indicates a conductive loss of 20 dB or more (true negative) or a severe sensorineural loss (false negative, because the 'hearing' nerve on the other side hears the sound by conduction through the skull).

10 Weber's test (Fig. 4) involves placing the vibrating tuning fork on the vertex or, alternatively, on the upper incisors, with opposing skull pressure applied, and asking the patient where the sound is coming from. With a conductive loss of 10 dB or more, the sound is heard in the affected ear, and with a sensorineural loss the sound is heard in the normal ear.

11 The postnasal space should be examined with a mirror or flexible nasoendoscope, although the examiners may not require you to actually carry this out.

12 The facial nerve should be examined, along with all the other cranial nerves if appropriate (for example in the case of a suspected acoustic neuroma). Any facial nerve abnormality should be graded according to the House–Brackmann scale.

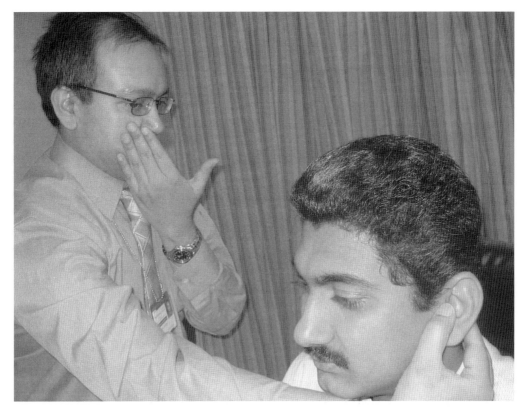

Fig. 2 Free speech hearing test

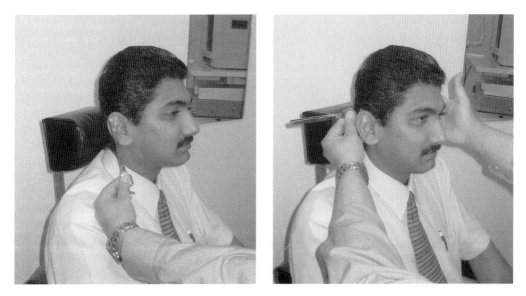

Fig. 3 (a, b) Rinne's test

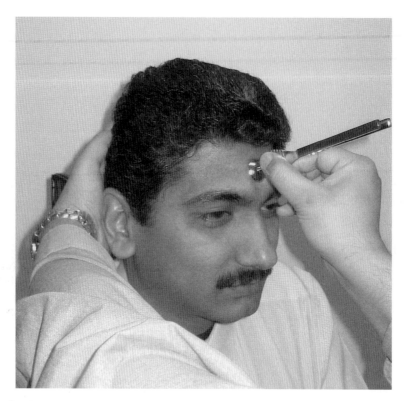

Fig. 4 Weber's test

Examination of the Nose

1 Introduce yourself to the patient and ask if any areas of the nose are tender.
2 Sit facing the patient, and fit your headlight. If using reflected light, position the lamp over the patient's left shoulder at head height. Sit with your knees together, and to the right of the patient's knees.
3 Examine the nose for symmetry from the front and the side. Note any scars, asymmetry, dorsal hump, tip depression, lateral deviation or rash.
4 Gently push the tip of the nose upwards and assess for columellar dislocation. Patency of the nasal airway may be assessed (Fig. 5) by asking the patient to close their mouth and breathe out onto a metal tongue depressor – note the condensation pattern. Alternatively, each nostril can be occluded in turn and the patient can try to sniff. Then watch the nasal vestibule for collapse as the patient takes a sniff in with both nostrils open.
5 Use a Thudichum speculum to open the nostril, assessing each nasal cavity in turn. Assess for septal deviation, mucosal health, septal perforation, polyps, and note any other pathology and its location. If there is septal deviation, try to distinguish whether it is cartilaginous (more anterior) or bony (posterior). A rigid or flexible scope may also be used for this assessment, although this is not usually required under exam conditions.

SECTION 3

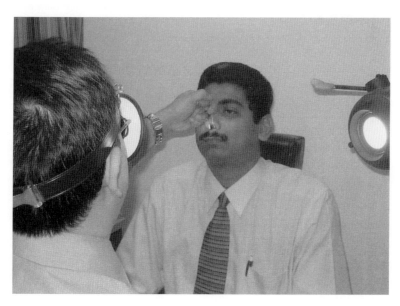

Fig. 5 Examination of the nasal passage

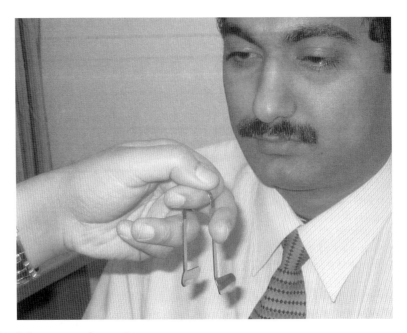

Fig. 6 Thudichum speculum grip

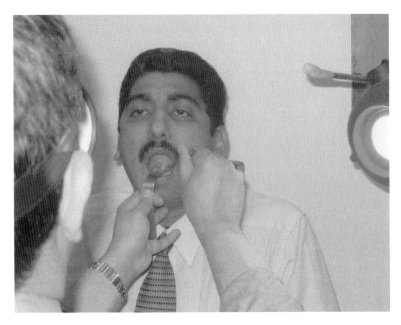

Fig. 7 Nasopharyngeal examination

A clearer view may be obtained by instilling a vasodilating solution or spray if the mucosa is congested, although this is in itself a significant finding. The patient may have to alter the tilt of their head for you to visualise the nasal airway from the floor to the roof. The speculum is generally held in the left hand as shown in Fig. 6, suspended from the index finger, with the blades controlled with the middle and ring fingers.

6   Inspect the oropharynx, the soft palate and the upper teeth, noting any abnormalities seen.

7   Look at the nasopharynx (Fig. 7), either with a warmed mirror with the tongue held with a tongue depressor, or with a flexible or rigid scope. This gives a view of the posterior ends of the septum and turbinates, the eustachian cushions and the fossae of Rosenmüller.

8   Inspect and palpate the neck, looking for lymphadenopathy – the anterior nose drains to the submandibular region and the posterior nose drains to the middle deep cervical nodes.

9   Mention to the examiner that you may want to assess olfactory function, perhaps by means of an olfactory testing kit.

Examination of the Throat

1 Introduce yourself to the patient and ask if any areas of the neck or throat are tender. Expose the patient's throat externally to the level of the clavicles.
2 Sit facing the patient, and fit your headlight. If using reflected light, position the lamp over the patient's left shoulder at head height. Sit with your knees together, and to the right of the patient's knees.
3 Note any obvious scars in the neck area or any tracheostomy or any asymmetry.
4 Ask the patient to open their mouth and inspect their oral cavity. Use two tongue depressors to examine the buccal mucosa on either side, the underside of the tongue and the floor of the mouth, the teeth and the parotid duct opening (Fig. 8). Examine the tonsils and posterior pharyngeal wall with only one depressor.
5 Use one gloved hand to palpate the base of the tongue and to bimanually palpate the submandibular duct for stones (Fig. 9).
6 Examine the postnasal space as before.

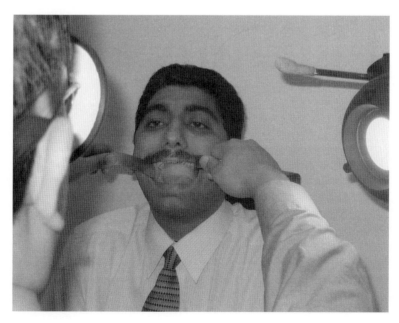

Fig. 8 Examination of the buccal mucosa

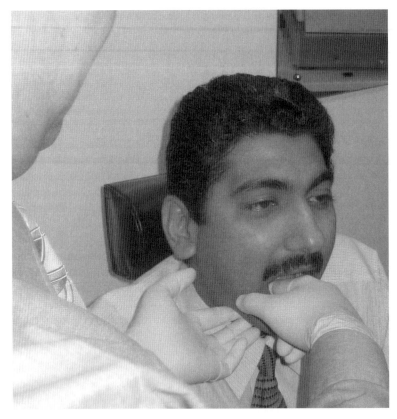

Fig. 9 Bimanual palpation of the submandibular gland

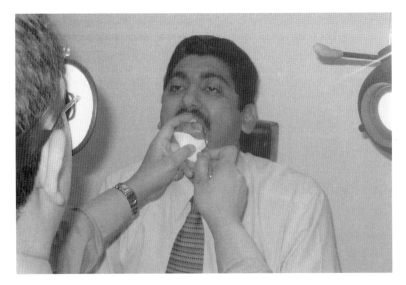

Fig. 10 Indirect laryngoscopy

7   Examine the larynx (Fig. 10) using either a warmed mirror with the patient's tongue held, or a flexible nasoendoscope. A good view should be obtained of the cords, epiglottis, valleculae, pyriform fossae, arytenoids and ventricular folds. This examination may not be necessary – you should be guided by the examiner.

8   Assess the patient's speech by getting them to count to ten, and assess their breathing by getting them to take a few deep breaths in and out. Ask them to swallow and watch the movement of the larynx.

9   Examine the neck as described on p. 239.

Examination of the Neck

1 Sit the patient on a chair with enough room to move behind. Expose the patient's neck to the level of the clavicles.

2 View the patient's neck from the front and the side, noting any scars, asymmetry or tracheostomy. If there is a visible lump, ask the patient to swallow to assess movement: this should be done by asking the patient to take a sip of water, hold it in their mouth and swallow it when required. Then ask the patient to open their mouth and stick their tongue out, in two separate movements. Note whether the lump moves with tongue protrusion.

3 Stand behind the patient and ask them to tilt their head slightly forwards to relax the neck muscles. Palpate the lymph node chains (Fig. 11) in a systematic fashion, eg start at the suprasternal notch, working up the midline to the trachea, thyroid and larynx, and then in the midline to the submental area, working back under the chin to the submandibular and jugulodigastric area, then down the anterior edge of the sterno-cleidomastoid to the clavicle. Assess for supra- and infraclavicular nodes. Move to the lower posterior edge of the sternocleidomastoid and work up to the angle of the jaw, the parotid gland, and the preauricular region, and then back to the mastoid, and down the anterior border of trapezius. Finish by palpating the occipital node area.

4 Any lump found should be assessed for size, consistency, fluctuance, mobility, pulsatility, tenderness, border, tethering to underlying or overlying structures, health of overlying skin or presence of a punctum, transillumination and bruit. It may be helpful when palpating a unilateral thyroid lump to hold the other side with the other hand.

5 If there is a lump in the parotid or submandibular area, use bimanual palpation to palpate the mass with one gloved hand. The facial nerve should be assessed in the case of a parotid lump.

6 If a lump is located in the thyroid region, then return to it and reassess for movement with swallowing and tongue protrusion while palpating it. Continue with auscultation for a thyroid bruit and percussion for retrosternal extension.

7 If a thyroid problem has been noted, or you have been asked to examine the thyroid gland, you should state to the examiners that you wish to examine the patient's thyroid status. This involves feeling the patient's hands for sweatiness, looking at the skin texture, and examining the pulse for abnormalities of rate or rhythm or irregularity. You should then look at the face for exophthalmos, lid retraction and chemosis. Assess eye movements and lid lag. Finally state that you would like to assess ankle reflexes.

8 If appropriate, ask the patient some questions relating to thyroid status:

♦ Are you on any thyroid medication?
♦ Have you had any thyroid operations?

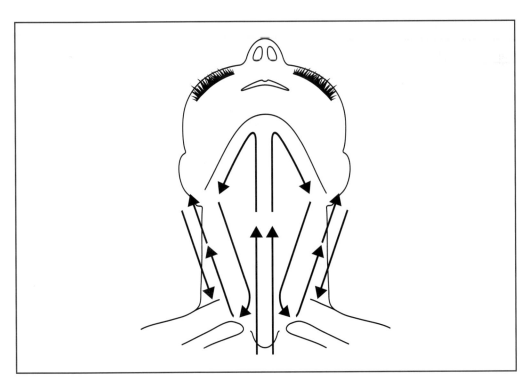

Fig. 11 Lymph node palpation

- Do you prefer a warm or a cold room?
- Have you lost or gained weight recently?
- Do you have diarrhoea or constipation?
- Do you have anxiety or depression?
- Have you had palpitations?
- Have your periods changed?
- Do you have any other medical problems?

SECTION

4

Clinical Scenarios

Clinical Scenarios

Part 2 of the DO-HNS examination includes one or more stations that involve taking a brief history from a patient (usually an actor) with an ENT problem. There may also be a station involving discussion of an operation or treatment, or obtaining consent for a particular ENT procedure.

This section presents some example scenarios with key questions to be asked and a brief discussion of the diagnosis. There is also a table listing common operations with their risks and complications.

1 Take a history from this lady who suffers from dizziness.

Key questions

◆ What exactly is the feeling you experience?
◆ Does the room spin?
◆ Is there any warning or 'aura'?
◆ How long does it last for?
◆ How often does it happen?
◆ Are there any precipitating or relieving factors?
◆ What other medical problems do you have?
◆ Is this problem getting worse?
◆ Was it sudden or gradual in onset?
◆ Was it accompanied by any other symptoms, such as tinnitus, hearing loss or upper respiratory tract symptoms?

The history should be taken in enough detail to establish whether true vertigo is present, and, if so, what the main cause is likely to be:

◆ Ménière's disease – episodes lasting a few minutes to hours, asymptomatic otherwise.
◆ Benign paroxysmal positional vertigo – exacerbated by particular movements, tends to get better with time, no tinnitus or hearing loss.
◆ Acute vestibulitis – may follow a viral infection, no tinnitus or hearing loss.

2 Take a history from this gentleman who suffers with nosebleeds.

Key questions

◆ Which nostril do you bleed from?
◆ Does the blood drip primarily from the front or the back?

- How often does it happen?
- How do you deal with episodes?
- How much blood do you lose?
- For how long have you been having nosebleeds?
- Have you recently suffered any trauma?
- Do you have any other medical problems, in particular hypertension?
- Are you on any medication?

The history should suggest where the bleeding comes from, what volume is lost, and what the precipitating cause might be. This information can then be used to determine the most appropriate treatment.

3 Take a history from this lady, whose young son suffers with recurrent throat infections.

Key questions

- How often does he get throat infections?
- How long do they last for?
- Is he able to eat or drink?
- Has he been treated with antibiotics?
- How long has he had this problem?
- Does he have any other medical problems?

The history should provide an indication of the severity and regularity of the infections, to help inform advice on whether the tonsils might need to be removed.

4 Take a history from this gentleman who has developed a hoarse voice.

Key questions

- What have you noticed has changed about your voice?
- How long have you had a hoarse voice for?
- Did it come on suddenly or gradually?
- Is your voice always hoarse or does it come and go?
- Does it ever 'go' completely?
- Is it getting worse?
- Does it get better when you rest your voice?
- What makes it worse?
- Are you a smoker?
- How much water do you drink?
- What is your job?
- Do you have any other medical problems?
- Have you had any recent operations or other interventions?

The history should establish the subjective perception of the voice – hoarseness may mean different things to different people. The pattern of hoarseness should be established.

Although voice abuse and poor vocal hygiene may not be the primary cause of pathology, improving these factors may help in treatment. High levels of smoking increase suspicion of a neoplastic lesion. Recent thyroid operations may be implicated in vocal cord immobility, and recent intubation may have caused trauma to the vocal cords.

INFORMATION ON COMMON ENT PROCEDURES

Table 1 gives common ENT procedures and the information that may need to be given to patients.

Procedure	Risks and complications	Hospital stay required	Time off work
Grommet insertion	Bleeding, infection, need for re-insertion	Day case	1–3 days
Adenoidectomy	Bleeding, pain, temporary voice change, damage to teeth	Overnight	1 week
Tonsillectomy	Bleeding, pain, temporary voice change, damage to teeth	Overnight	1–2 weeks
Manipulation of fractured nasal bone	Bleeding, pain, need for a splint or cast, no improvement possible, need for septorhinoplasty	Day case	3–5 days
Septoplasty	Bleeding, discomfort from packs, possible resultant deformity	Overnight	1–2 weeks
Septorhinoplasty	Bleeding, discomfort from nasal packing, periorbital haematomas, possibly no improvement or even deterioration, need to wear plaster cast	Overnight	2 weeks
Myringoplasty	Bleeding, infection, scar, damage to hearing, damage to facial nerve/chorda tympani, failure of graft, discomfort from ear pack	Overnight	1 week
Mastoidectomy	Infection, scar, damage to hearing, damage to facial nerve/chorda tympani, vertigo, need to repeat procedure if disease not eradicated, need for a drain	Overnight	2 weeks
Superficial parotidectomy	Bleeding, scar, infection, damage to facial nerve/ greater auricular nerve, recurrence possible, Frey's syndrome	Overnight	2 weeks
Radical neck dissection	Bleeding, infection, scar, damage to great vessels, damage to vagus/phrenic/hypoglossal/axillary nerves, damage to sternocleidomastoid muscle, drain	3–5 days	2–4 weeks
Functional endoscopic sinus surgery (FESS)	Bleeding, nasal packing, damage to orbital contents, CSF leak, recurrence of pathology	1–2 days	2 weeks
Thyroidectomy	Bleeding, scar, infection, airway compromise, damage to RLN, voice change, calcium derangement, need for thyroxine supplementation	1–3 days	2 weeks

Table 1 Summary of common ENT procedures

SECTION 4

OSCE Questions

This section gives examples of Objective Structured Clinical Examination questions, followed by a brief explanation of the correct answer. We have attempted to reproduce clinical photographs with sufficient detail to enable you to attempt an answer. Answers to OSCEs should be brief and unambiguous; do not spend time writing a miniature essay. For further practice, use a picture book on ENT.

OSCE Questions

OSCE Station 1: Question

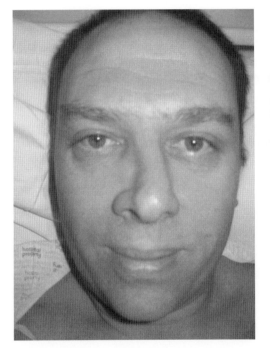 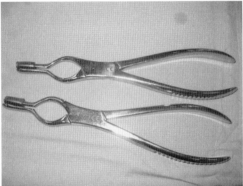

A   This patient sustained a traumatic blow to the nose. What is the diagnosis?

B   What are the options for treatment?

C   If the patient is left untreated, what risks should he be aware of?

D   Name this piece of equipment (two shown in the figure) and describe its use.

OSCE Station 1: Answer

A This patient has a fracture of the nasal bone and may also have a traumatic dislocation of the nasal cartilage.

B If he is seen immediately after the incident, it may be possible to realign the nasal bone immediately. Failing this, he will require an ENT opinion at 7–10 days, once the swelling has receded, but before the nasal bone itself has set. This gives an opportunity to manipulate the fracture, either under local anaesthetic or, more usually, under general anaesthetic. The surgeon attempts to reduce the fracture by pressure on the nose and the use of reduction equipment such as Walshingham's forceps (see figure). A cast may be necessary to keep the nose in position, or it may be necessary to use nasal splints if the nasal septum is dislocated.

C Untreated nasal fractures may result in immediate septal haematomas and bleeding, which may require urgent treatment. In the longer term, nasal obstruction may result, along with unacceptable cosmesis for the patient. This may require an operation in the future to correct the defect, such as a septorhinoplasty, which carries its own risks of failure.

D Walshingham's forceps – these are used with one blade inside the nasal passageway and the other on the external skin, to grip different parts of the nasal bone and adjust their alignment.

OSCE Station 2: Question

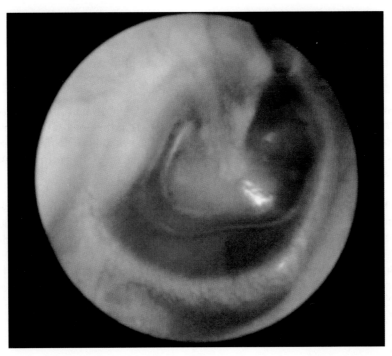

The figure shows otitis media with effusion, or glue ear. A fluid level is clearly visible.

A   Describe the audiogram you would get for this ear in this patient.

B   What type of tympanogram would you get for this patient?

C   Describe the surgical procedure that is indicated for this condition.

D   What is the aetiology of this problem?

OSCE Station 2: Answer

A   A pure tone audiogram is likely to show a conductive hearing loss of the order of 20–40 dB.

B   A tympanogram is likely to show a type B picture, ie a flat tympanogram, indicating low compliance.

C   Grommet insertion involves a myringoplasty in the antero-inferior, or postero-inferior portion of the ear canal. Then a grommet is inserted in this area, which may be of the Shah or Shepherd type. These grommets are self-extruding and on average stay in for 9 months. T-tubes may be used in cases of persistent glue ear, although they are associated with a high rate of persistent perforation.

D   Eustachian tube dysfunction, common in younger children, perhaps due to the immature anatomy and large adenoids, leads to difficulty equalising the pressure between the postnasal space and middle ear. This causes an enclosed middle ear air space, and respiratory tissue lining this space uses oxygen and hence creates a vacuum. Fluid is drawn from the surrounding tissue to form the 'glue', which is of high protein content and may contain mucopolysaccharides, white cells, epithelial cells and blood.

OSCE Station 3: Question

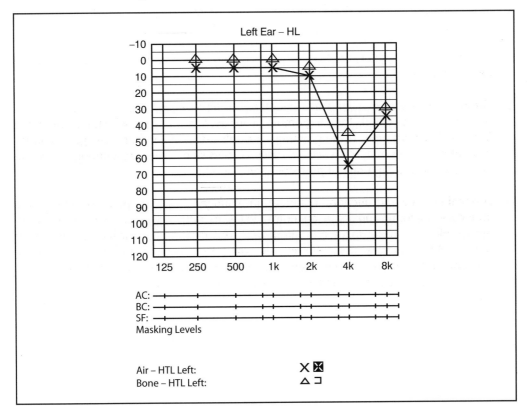

A patient has the audiogram shown, and the right ear shows an identical picture.

A Describe the audiogram. What is the diagnosis?

B Explain what causes the audiogram shown.

C If the right ear had a **normal** audiogram, what would the differential diagnosis be?

OSCE Station 3: Answer

A The audiogram shows a sensorineural hearing loss specifically at 4 kHz, which is the picture classically associated with noise-induced hearing loss. The patient should be questioned about previous exposure to loud noise, and if exposure is continuing, should be advised about the use of ear defenders to protect the ears against further damage.

B The fact that the 4 kHz frequency is most affected is thought to be due to the fact that the cochlea is most sensitive to noises at this frequency, and hence sounds at this frequency have the greatest potential for causing stress to the basilar membrane.

C A normal audiogram on the contralateral side may simply indicate that the subject has been exposed to unilateral noise, for example due to firing a rifle. However, any case of unilateral sensorineural deafness should be investigated for evidence of an acoustic neuroma (vestibular schwannoma), and this may involve an MRI scan of the internal auditory meatus to look for a growth on the acoustic nerve.

OSCE Station 4: Question

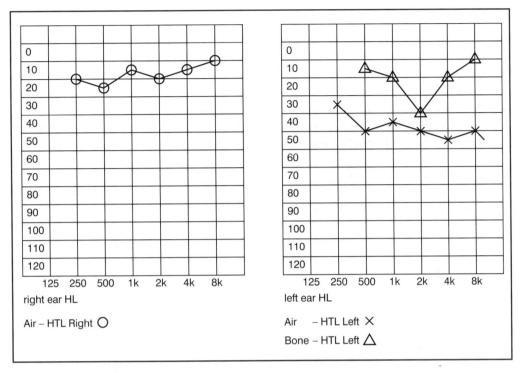

A What does the audiogram of the female patient in the figure show?

B What is the most likely diagnosis?

C If the patient were contemplating pregnancy, would you advise her to have treatment before or after pregnancy?

OSCE Station 4: Answer

A   This audiogram shows a unilateral conductive defect, with a bone conduction dip at 2 kHz.

B   This picture is characteristic of otosclerosis, and this is known as 'Carhart's notch'. The incidence of otosclerosis in both sexes is equal, and it is inherited as an autosomal dominant condition.

C   Otosclerosis is known to worsen during pregnancy, and for this reason it is better that the patient should start her family before treatment is considered for the condition, as it may recur in subsequent pregnancies.

OSCE Station 5: Question

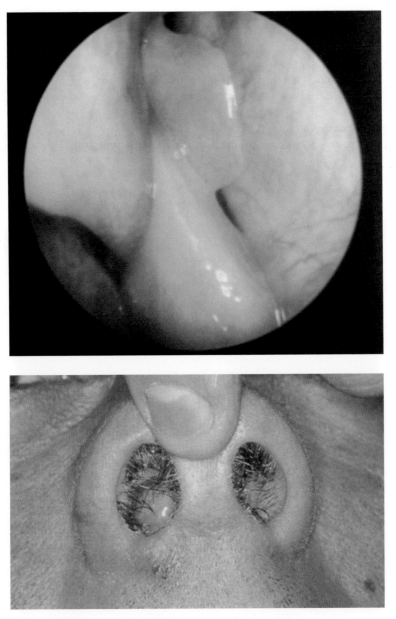

A   What is shown in the figures and what is the diagnosis?

B   What treatment is appropriate, and what risks should be mentioned?

OSCE Station 5: Answer

A   The figures show an internal view and an external view of the nasal cavity. There is a nasal polyp present. Nasal polyps represent prolapse of the nasal mucosa, either from the maxillary sinus area or from the ethmoid sinus area. They may grow to obstruct the nasal airway. Unilateral polyps, or any form of unilateral sinus pathology should be carefully investigated, as neoplastic disease may present with unilateral symptoms. However, the appearance here is characteristic of benign nasal polyposis.

B   Treatment is by nasal polypectomy, usually carried out these days by functional endoscopic sinus surgery (FESS). Risks that should be mentioned include:

◆   risks of general anaesthesia
◆   risk of damage to the eyes and eye muscles
◆   bleeding from the nose and the need for pack insertion
◆   periorbital haematoma
◆   and polyp recurrence postoperatively.

Conservative treatment may also be considered in the form of topical nasal steroid treatment, although once polyps have reached this size it is largely irrelevant.

OSCE Station 6: Question

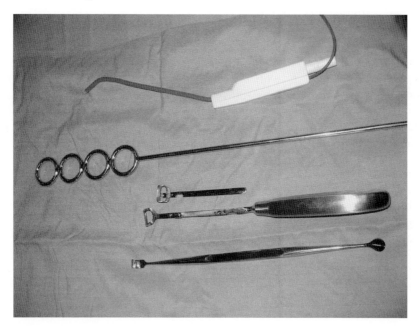

A   Name these instruments and briefly describe their use.

B   What operation are they used for?

C   Name two other instruments used in this operation.

OSCE Station 6: Answer

A From above downwards:

- Suction diathermy – used for directly cauterising adenoid tissue.
- Draffin rod – for supporting the Boyle–Davis gag in a pair during the procedure.
- Barhill adenoid curette with guard – for curetting adenoidal tissue. The guard enables it to be used more effectively when the tissue is overly corrugated.
- Mollinson's pillar retractor – for retracting the tonsillar pillars and tongue base to access bleeding points.

B These instruments are used in adenotonsillectomy.

C Other instruments used include an angled mirror, Gwynne–Evans tonsil dissectors, Dennis–Brown forceps, Negus knot pusher, Negus clamp, Wilson clamp and Eve tonsil snare.

OSCE Station 7: Question

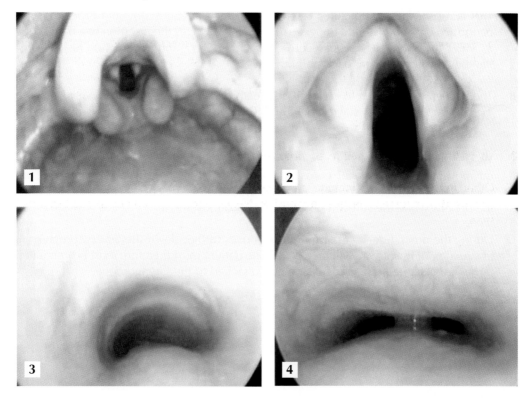

A   These pictures were taken during a procedure under anaesthesia. Describe what anatomical areas are shown.

B   What is the most obvious pathology shown in these pictures?

C   If the patient was woken from anaesthesia while the top left view was monitored, what information might be gained?

D   How is the patient ventilated during this procedure?

OSCE Station 7: Answer

A This is a series of four pictures taken from a microlaryngoscopy and bronchoscopy, performed on a young child under anaesthesia. It involves the insertion of a rigid scope to view the larynx (1), vocal cords (2), trachea (3) and carina (4), respectively. Photographs are taken at each point.

B The trachea can be seen to collapse on breathing, narrowing the airway, especially in the bottom right image, suggesting a high degree of tracheomalacia. This may require a laryngotracheal reconstruction if it presents a threat to the child's health.

C Waking the patient while the camera is in the top left position would give information on movement of the vocal cords, especially whether there is any degree of cord paralysis or paradoxical cord movement with breathing (the anaesthetist usually counts the breaths while the surgeon observes the cord movement).

D During the procedure, as the rigid scope moves further down the airway, progressive obstruction of the airway will take place. The patient must therefore must be ventilated through the scope itself, using a side port attached to the laryngoscope.

OSCE Station 8: Question

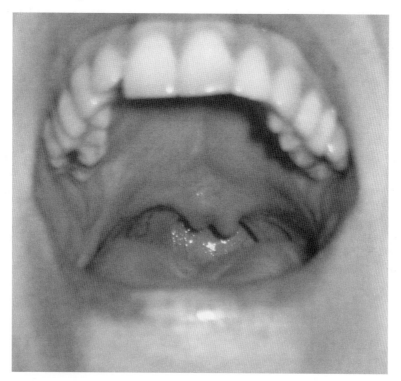

A What congenital abnormality is shown in the figure?

B What other associated abnormality may be present on examination?

C What common operation may be contraindicated?

OSCE Station 8: Answer

A   The figure shows a bifid uvula, formed due to incomplete fusion of the soft palate.

B   In itself, it is an inconsequential finding, but it may be associated with incomplete fusion of the underlying maxillary processes. This may have been fully covered with mucous membrane, leading to a submucous cleft.

C   This defect, like a full-thickness cleft, is a contraindication to adenoidectomy due to the risk of consequent hypernasal speech.

OSCE Station 9: Question

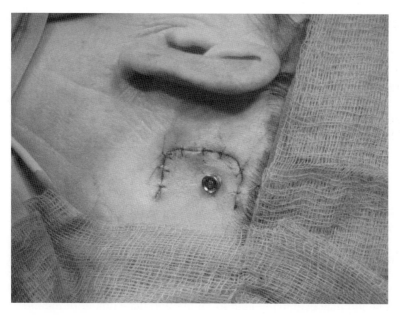

A   What is shown in the figure?

B   How is this attachment used?

C   In what situations might it be indicated?

D   What are the risks?

SECTION 5

OSCE Station 9: Answer

A The figure shows an abutment for a bone-anchored hearing aid (BAHA) fitted behind the ear.

B It can be inserted under local or general anaesthetic, and involves a split-skin or full-thickness skin graft. A titanium abutment is then fixed to the skull after drilling, using a mechanical device which applies a fixed torque to the screw thread. The abutment is then used to fit an aid, which vibrates in response to detected sound and transmits vibrations through the skull to the auditory nerve.

C A BAHA may be indicated in cases of single-sided deafness, when cross-transmission of bone-conducted sound acts as a hearing substitute for the deaf ear. It also may be useful when hearing aids are not tolerated or contraindicated, for example in cases of microtia where there is no suitable attachment point for the aid, or where an in-the-ear hearing aid causes infection or discharge.

D Risks of the procedure include infection, scar, and numbness over the skin, and there is a long-term risk of infection at the site which is why patients are given strict instructions to keep the site meticulously clean. Infection may cause problems with loosening and may eventually lead to failure and detachment of the aid.

OSCE Station 10: Question

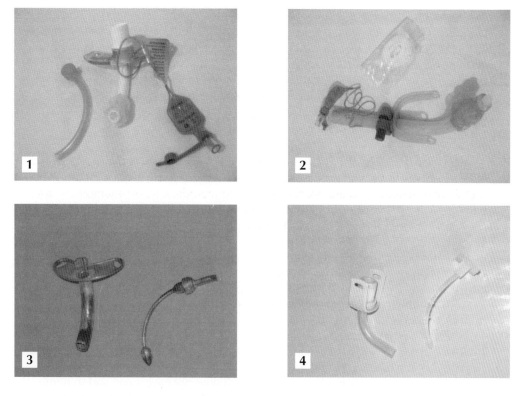

A   Briefly describe the procedure of tracheostomy insertion.

B   What are the indications for a tracheostomy?

C   Name the tracheostomy tubes shown and discuss situations in which they might be used.

SECTION 5

OSCE Station 10: Answer

A   Tracheostomy insertion is usually performed under general anaesthetic. The patient is placed in a neck-extended position, and a horizontal incision is made halfway between the suprasternal notch and the cricoid. Blunt dissection is carried out in the midline through the subcutaneous fat and pretracheal fascia. The strap muscles are retracted and the thyroid isthmus is either retracted or divided to expose the trachea. This is then incised between the second and fourth tracheal rings and the tracheostomy tube inserted.

B   Indications for tracheostomy include:

◆   Mechanical obstruction – neoplasia, trauma, recurrent laryngeal nerve paralysis, inflammation.
◆   Protection of the airway – in patients who are prone to aspiration due to paralysis or neurological disease.
◆   Reduction in dead space – to optimise airflow in patients requiring long-term ventilation.

C   1   This is a cuffed fenestrated tube, which is used in medium- to long-term tracheostomy care when the patient requires a voice.
   2   This is an cuffed adjustable flange tube, used when a distal airway obstruction needs to be bypassed.
   3   This is a silver Negus tube, and it is indicated when long-term tracheostomy is required in patients with thin necks.
   4   This is a paediatric tracheostomy tube, which does not have a cuff and so minimises trauma to the trachea.

OSCE Station 11: Question

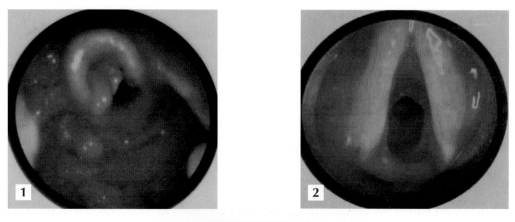

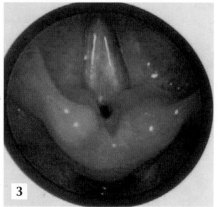

Describe the laryngeal pathologies shown.

OSCE Station 11: Answer

1 Laryngeal papillomatosis – this is a self-limiting condition, which usually recedes with time, although treatment to remove the papillomas or even a tracheostomy may be necessary in severe cases.

2 Subglottic stenosis – most commonly caused by the effects of long-term intubation and consequent trauma to the larynx. Laryngotracheal reconstruction may be necessary to widen the lumen of the airway.

3 Laryngeal web – this is a congenital abnormality which obstructs the airway, but which may be treated by laser breakdown of the web.

OSCE Station 12: Question

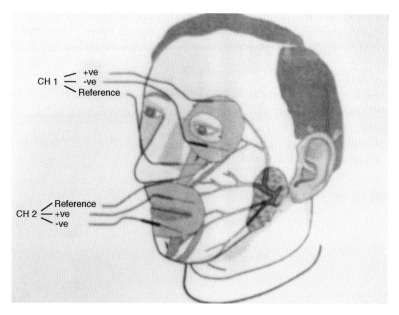

A   What piece of equipment is shown in the diagram?

B   In what situations might it be used?

OSCE Station 12: Answer

A   The diagram shows the positioning for facial nerve monitoring equipment, used to monitor the upper and lower divisions of the facial nerve. The leads shown are connected to a monitor unit, which alerts the operator when the nerve is touched or disturbed.

B   This equipment may be useful in certain operations when the nerve is at risk, such as:

   ◆ parotid surgery
   ◆ cerebellopontine angle tumour surgery
   ◆ mastoid surgery.

It can only be used when neuromuscular blockade is not present.

OSCE Station 13: Question

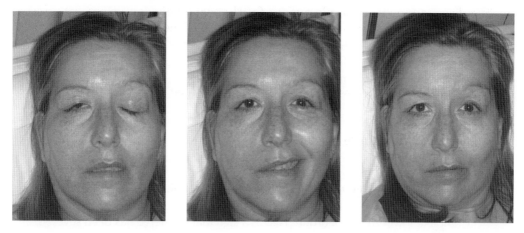

The patient shown has been asked to close her eyes, to smile, and to raise her eyebrows.

A   On which side is the pathology evident?

B   How can this be graded, and what is the grade shown in this patient?

C   List three possible diagnoses and outline for each the treatment that may be required.

OSCE Station 13: Answer

A   The patient has evident right facial nerve palsy.

B   This is graded using the House–Brackmann grading system (see page 114). This patient displays incomplete eye closure, slight mouth movement and no forehead movement, giving her a House–Brackmann grading of IV or V.

C   Possible diagnoses are:

- Bell's palsy – a diagnosis of exclusion in 55% of cases. It may be a virally induced response and is treated with steroids, aciclovir, artificial tears and eye patches.
- Ramsay Hunt syndrome – present in 7% and caused by herpes zoster virus. Vesicles may be seen in the external ear canal. Aciclovir 800 mg five times a day may help.
- Trauma – present in 19%. This may be associated with a temporal bone fracture. Complete lower motor neurone palsy is a sign that the nerve has been severed, and exploration is indicated.
- Tumour – in 6%. May originate in the parotid or from the nerve itself. The tumour may require surgical removal, and a graft to replace the infiltrated portion may be required.
- Ear infection – in 4%. Acute or chronic otitis media and malignant otitis externa may cause palsy and exploration of the mastoid may be indicated, although in simple acute otitis media a conservative approach is employed.

OSCE Station 14: Question

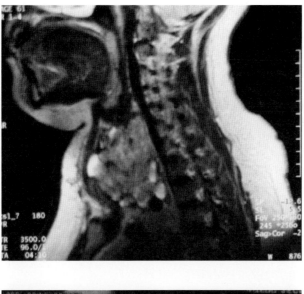

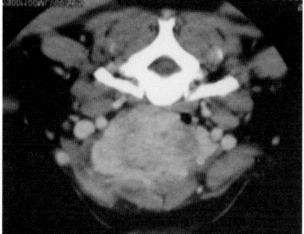

Two views of a patient's neck are shown.

A What investigations are shown? Name two clinical signs that may be present. .

B The lump shown was removed under general anaesthetic. Upon waking up, the patient had stridor, and was re-anaesthetised and given a tracheostomy. What is the explanation for the stridor?

C Postoperatively the patient developed tingling in her fingers. What is the reason for this and what clinical sign may be present? What treatment is indicated?

OSCE Station 14: Answer

A   A sagittal MRI and axial CT section of a patient's neck are shown. This is a large thyroid mass, due to a papillary carcinoma. The mass can be seen to be compressing and deviating the trachea, and may cause breathlessness and stridor, cosmetic deformity, problems with swallowing, and thyroid function abnormalities. Pressure effects on other surrounding structures, such as the carotid artery and jugular vein, may occur.

B   The patient underwent total thyroidectomy, and waking stridor shows that there was some damage to both RLNs, leaving the vocal cords fixed in a paramedian position. Air entry was possible but a tracheostomy was advisable to make the airway safe.

C   The patient needed postoperative measurements of calcium concentration daily, due to the fact that the parathyroid glands may have been injured during the operation. Tingling fingers suggests hypocalcaemia, and Chvostek's sign (a shooting facial pain on tapping just anterior to the parotid gland) may be present. Replacement with alfacalcidol and calcium may be indicated.

OSCE Station 15: Question

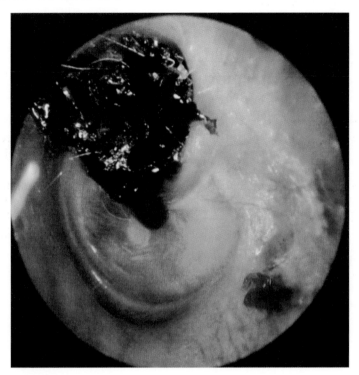

A   What is the diagnosis?

B   What are the two commonest symptoms?

C   What operation is necessary?

OSCE Station 15: Answer

A   The figure shows a cholesteatoma breaking through the tympanic membrane, with some keratin visible in the canal and opacity behind the membrane.

B   ◆ Hearing loss, which may be sensorineural (due to the effects of toxins on the hearing nerves), conductive (due to the effect of ossicular destruction), or mixed.
   ◆ Discharge from the ear, which may be reported as foul-smelling, creamy.
   ◆ Dizziness is not common, but may signify a labyrinthine fistula.

C   A mastoidectomy would provide the best definitive treatment, and the best chance of avoiding recurrence. It would be accompanied by tympanoplasty. Mastoidectomies may be classified as:

   ◆ Cortical mastoidectomy – the mastoid cortex is drilled out through a postauricular incision, leaving the posterior canal wall intact.
   ◆ Modified radical mastoidectomy – the canal wall is removed, either through an approach from the front or behind from the mastoid cortex.
   ◆ Combined-approach tympanoplasty – a cortical mastoidectomy is extended posteriorly to visualise the middle ear via a posterior tympanotomy.

OSCE Station 16: Question

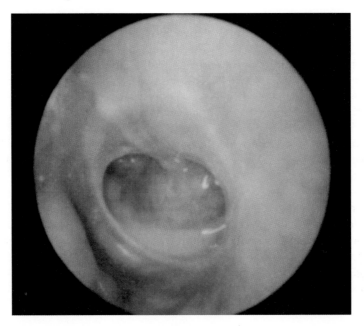

A   What is the diagnosis?

B   Name five potential complications of this disease.

OSCE Station 16: Answer

A This is chronic suppurative otitis media (CSOM), with a chronic perforation and discharge. The perforation in this case seems to be tubotympanic.

B Complications include:

- otitis externa
- ossicular damage
- sensorineural hearing loss
- vertigo
- tympanosclerosis
- adhesions.

If attico-antral CSOM is present, further possible complications include facial nerve palsy, carcinoma of the middle ear, labyrinthine fistula, lateral sinus thrombosis, meningitis, and extradural/subdural/intracerebral abscesses.

OSCE Station 17: Question

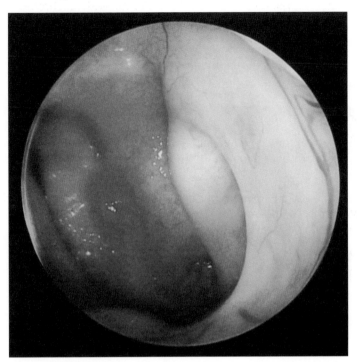

A   What area are we looking at?

B   Which part would you take a biopsy from in a case of unilateral glue ear?

C   With a carcinoma in this area, what complications could manifest?

OSCE Station 17: Answer

A   The left eustachian tube cushion area of the nasopharynx, via a nasoendoscopic view.

B   The suspicion is of a nasopharyngeal tumour, which usually arises in the fossa of Rosenmüller, and this would be the ideal biopsy site.

C   Glue ear, as mentioned, is common, and is due to anterior spread to the eustachian tube. Posterior spread to the parapharyngeal space may cause mandibular nerve paralysis and trismus. Spread to the retrostyloid space produces IX–XII nerve palsies and involvement of the cervical chain, causing Horner's syndrome. Spread superiorly may cause cranial nerve paralysis (III/IV/V), leading to diplopia, facial numbness or headaches.

OSCE Station 18: Question

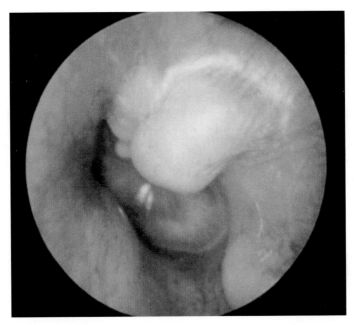

A What can be seen in this ear canal?

B How would you manage this patient?

OSCE Station 18: Answer

A   This is an exostosis, which is a benign over-development of bone in the external ear canal. It seems to be caused by a reaction to cold water in the ear and is quite common in deep sea divers.

B   If the patient is asymptomatic, it may be prudent to proceed conservatively. However, if the canal is blocked or there is infection, hearing loss or build-up of debris as a result of the exostosis, surgical removal is indicated. This may be via an endoaural or a post-aural approach.

OSCE Station 19: Question

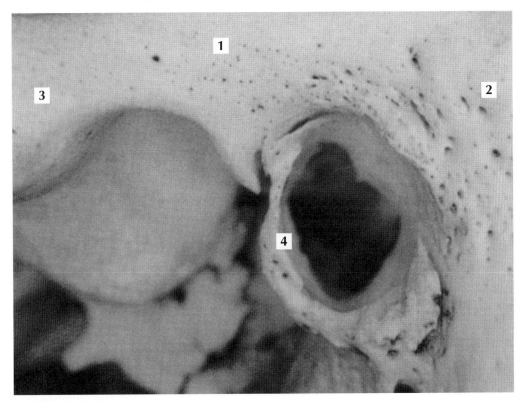

A   Name the parts of the bones labelled 1, 2, 3 and 4.

B   What foramen does the facial nerve exit from?

OSCE Station 19: Answer

A **1** Squamous portion of the temporal bone
   2 Petrous portion of the temporal bone
   3 Zygomatic arch of temporal bone
   4 Tympanic ring of temporal bone

B The facial nerve gives off fibres to the chorda tympani and the stapedius muscle, and then exits from the stylomastoid foramen of the temporal bone, after which it divides into its five branches.

OSCE Station 20: Question

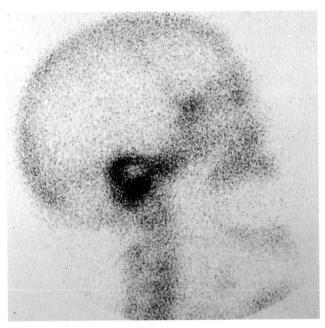

A This bone scan is of an elderly patient with diabetes. What is the diagnosis?

B Which organism is responsible for this condition and what is the antibiotic of choice to treat it?

C Name three complications of this disease.

OSCE Station 20: Answer

A   This bone scan shows malignant otitis externa.

B   Malignant otitis externa is a necrotising inflammation which largely occurs in people with diabetes. It is caused by *Pseudomonas aeruginosa* and is treated with ciprofloxacin, although this therapy should be modified in the light of any culture results obtained.

C   The infection may spread through the cartilaginous meatus, and deep into the retro-mandibular fossa, along the base of the skull to the jugular foramen. Palsies of cranial nerves VII–XII may result, as well as sigmoid sinus thrombosis, intracranial abscesses and meningitis.

OSCE Station 21: Question

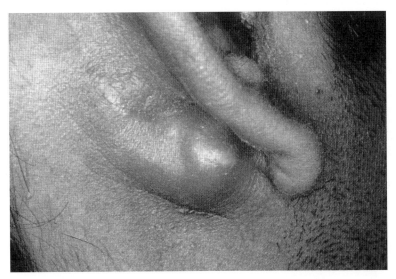

A   This man presented unwell, with fever, hearing loss and otalgia. What is the likely diagnosis?

B   What investigation is indicated?

C   What is the surgical treatment?

OSCE Station 21: Answer

A This is acute mastoiditis, with a fluctuant, tender postauricular area over the mastoid bone, along with discharge and a protruding ear. It represents a failure of resolution of otitis media and an extension of infection into the middle ear, causing a subperiosteal abscess.

B A CT scan is indicated to investigate the degree of inflammation in the mastoid bone.

C Mastoid exploration and eradication of disease is necessary to treat this condition.

OSCE Station 22: Question

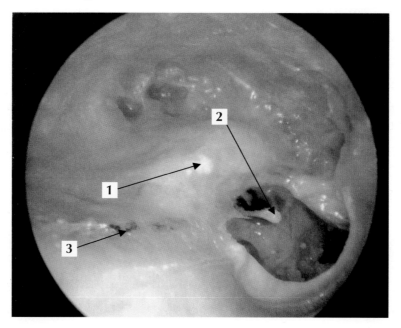

A What operation has this patient had?

B Name structures 1, 2 and 3.

OSCE Station 22: Answer

A This patient has had a radical mastoidectomy.

B 1 Facial nerve ridge, protecting facial nerve
    2 Head of the stapes bone
    3 Venous sigmoid sinus

OSCE Station 23: Question

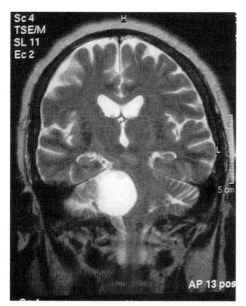 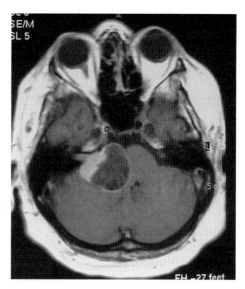

A   In these MRI scans, what is the most likely diagnosis?

B   In bilateral cases, what condition is usually associated with this?

C   If this patient had facial palsy, which classification scheme would you use to grade the
palsy clinically?

OSCE Station 23: Answer

A   Acoustic neuroma.

B   Neurofibromatosis type 2, which is an autosomal dominant disease caused by a mutation in chromosome 22.

C   The palsy can be graded using the House–Brackmann grading scheme (see page 114) in which I is normal movement and VI is total paralysis.

OSCE Station 24: Question

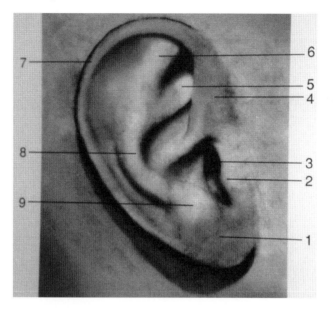

A Name parts 1–9 in the figure.

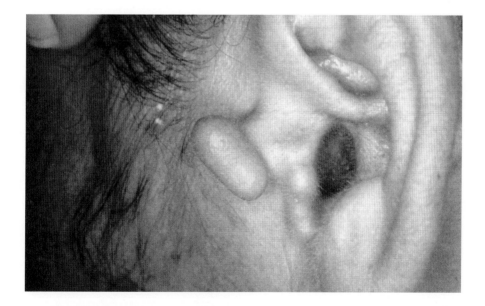

B What are the indications for surgical correction in the condition shown above?

OSCE Station 24: Answer

A **1** Lobe
    2 Tragus
    3 External auditory meatus
    4 Crus helicis
    5 Crus anthelicis
    6 Crus anthelicis
    7 Helix
    8 Antihelix
    9 Antitragus

B The figure shows an accessory auricle, formed by incomplete closure of the first branchial cleft or failure of fusion of the auricular hillocks of His. It may be associated with an aural fistula. Indications for surgery are cosmesis, persistent discharge, swelling or infection of a preauricular fistula, bearing in mind that there is a risk of damage to the facial nerve or parotid gland.

OSCE Station 25: Question

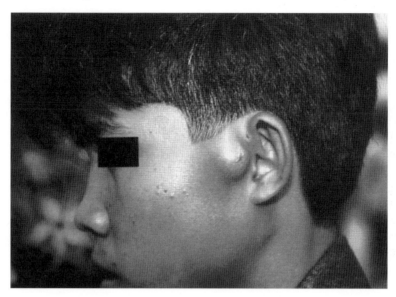

A   What is the diagnosis?

B   What is the treatment?

SECTION 5

OSCE Station 25: Answer

A   This is an infected preauricular sinus, with a swelling visible in the preauricular area and a fistula punctum visible on the ascending helix. It is caused by failure of fusion of auricular hillocks or incomplete closure of the first branchial cleft.

B   Acute treatment should include antibiotics and pain relief, with therapy tailored to results of swabs taken from the discharge from the sinus. At a later stage, excision of the sinus is indicated, with methylene blue dye injected in the punctum to outline the extent of the sinus. All the branches of the sinus tract are then excised carefully, taking care not to damage the facial nerve.

OSCE Station 26: Question

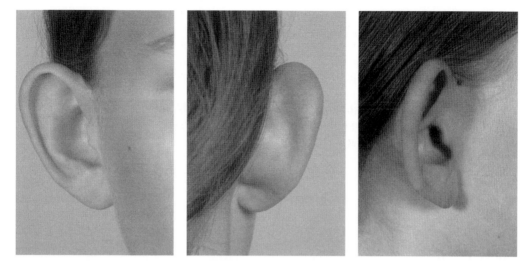

A   What is absent in these three views of the same ear?

B   What is the ideal age for surgical correction, and why?

C   Name three risks of pinnaplasty surgery.

OSCE Station 26: Answer

A   The antihelix is absent, leading to a failure of folding of the ear cartilage and consequent protrusion.

B   The operation should be carried out in the pre-school years, so that the child is not subject to teasing from his or her peers.

C   ◆ Perichondrial haematoma, leading to destruction of cartilage.
     ◆ Asymmetrical result, leading to poor cosmetic appearance.
     ◆ Stenosis of the ear canal.

OSCE Station 27: Question

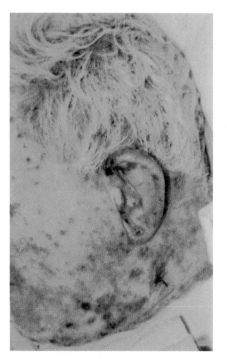

A   Name the abnormality shown in the figure.

B   What treatment would you offer this patient (who has good hearing)?

C   Where else in the body might the same process occur?

OSCE Station 27: Answer

A This shows herpes zoster, commonly known as shingles. When the geniculate ganglion is affected this is known as Ramsay Hunt syndrome.

B Treatment should include pain relief and aciclovir, with follow-up and vitamins if necessary.

C Any dermatome in the skin may be involved in the process, which represents a reactivation of dormant herpes zoster infection.

OSCE Station 28: Question

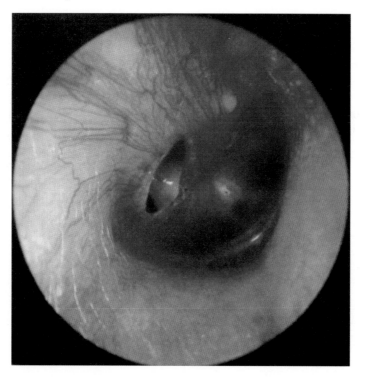

A   Describe what you can see.

B   What are the treatment options in this patient, who has mild conductive deafness?

OSCE Station 28: Answer

A This is a traumatic perforation of the tympanic membrane, with no associated infection visible.

B If the perforation is recent, conservative treatment should be the first line, with reassessment of hearing and the membrane after a few months. Most perforations heal themselves in the absence of any underlying disease. However, persistent perforation with hearing loss or persistent discharge may be considered for treatment by myringoplasty.

OSCE Station 29: Question

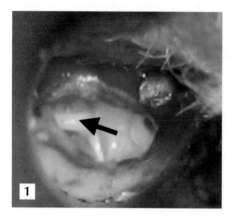

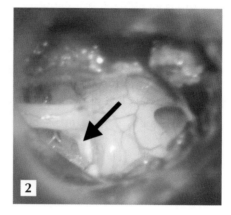

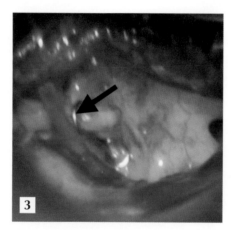

The three pictures shown describe three successive stages of an operation.

A   What is the arrowed structure visible in picture 1?

B   What is the arrowed structure that has been severed in picture 2?

C   What is the arrowed metal structure visible in picture 3?

D   What operation is being performed?

E   What risks should the patient be informed of before this procedure?

OSCE Station 29: Answer

A   The long process of the incus, which attaches to the head of the stapes underneath.

B   The stapedius tendon.

C   A metal stapes prosthesis, which has been hooked onto the long process of the incus, and whose body has been attached to the remainder of the stapes footplate.

D   This sequence of pictures is of a stapedectomy.

E   Risks of stapedectomy include:

  ◆ deafness
  ◆ perilymph fistula
  ◆ injury to the chorda tympani/facial nerve
  ◆ prosthesis detachment
  ◆ necrosis of the incus.

OSCE Station 30: Question

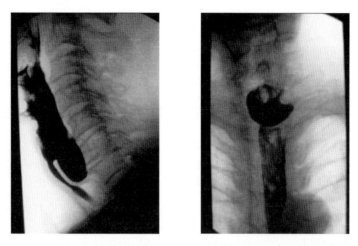

A These pictures are taken from a barium swallow sequence. What pathology is shown?

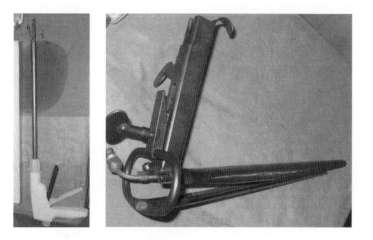

B These figures show equipment used in the treatment of this condition. What procedure uses this equipment?

C Apart from those common to any general anaesthetic procedure, name two complications that may arise from this procedure.

OSCE Station 30: Answer

A   A large pharyngeal pouch.

B   This is a stapling gun and bivalve oesophagoscopes, used in endoscopic stapling of pharyngeal pouches. The bivalve scope is inserted, with the lower blade in the pouch, and the upper, longer blade in the lumen of the oesophagus. This then presents the cricopharyngeal 'bar' as a target for the staple gun, which is passed across the bar and fired. The bar is divided by this action, with staples left on each side to prevent air leakage and mediastinitis.

C   The endoscopic stapling procedure is a very convenient way to treat patients when it is successful. However there is potential for serious complications:

*   The oesophagus may be perforated if the gun or scope are pushed too far into the pouch.
*   The teeth may be damaged in the process of manoeuvring the scope or gun.
*   The larynx or vocal cords may be damaged.
*   The problem may not be cured by the operation, and may recur even after a successful procedure (10% is the recurrence rate usually quoted).

OSCE Station 31: Question

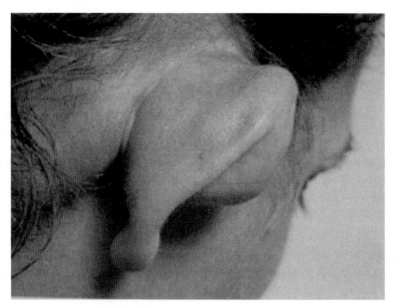

A   Describe what is shown in the figure.

B   What treatment is indicated, and what are the consequences if it is not carried out?

C   Where else in the body might the same process occur that might also be treated by an otolaryngologist?

SECTION 5

OSCE Station 31: Answer

A   The figure shows a periauricular haematoma. This is a collection of blood in the perichondrial area, which leads to dissection of the skin and perichondrial layer from the pinna cartilage, and so may cause necrosis of that cartilage.

B   Urgent drainage of a periauricular haematoma is required, ideally involving the suturing of a dressing around the area, and application of pressure to the pinna to prevent re-collection of haematoma. Failure to prevent re-collection may lead to sclerosis of the cartilage and the characteristic 'cauliflower ear' appearance.

C   This process may also occur if there is a haematoma on both sides of the nasal cartilage, leading to elevation of the mucoperiosteum from its cartilaginous attachment. Unless this is drained there may be a consequent death of the septal cartilage and resultant perforation.

OSCE Station 32: Question

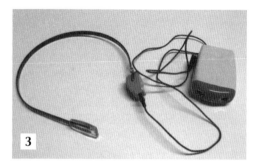

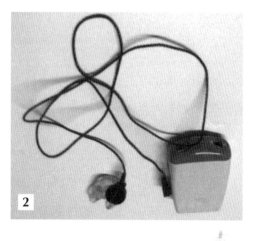

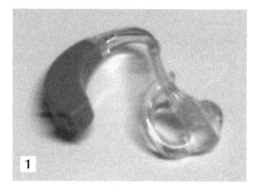

A Name the hearing aids shown, and a situation in which each one might be appropriate.

B The hearing aid shown in (1) has three settings, labelled O, T and M. What do these mean?

OSCE Station 32: Answer

A **1** Behind-the-ear – useful for mild to moderate presbycusis, where there is some useful hearing that may be amplified.

2 On-the-body – severe presbycusis that requires powerful amplification.

3 Bone-conduction – useful when occlusion of the external ear canal leads to problems with infection, or when external ear stenosis is present.

B **O** – Off

T – Television or telephone induction coil

M – Microphone (for normal use)

OSCE Station 33: Question

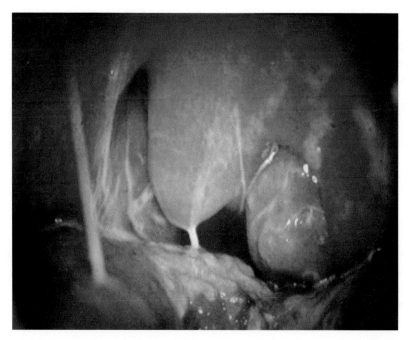

A This patient has a diagnosis of tonsillitis. What other feature is seen on the figure?

B Name three symptoms the patient might complain of.

C Name three treatments that might be helpful in this case.

D Name three complications that may arise.

OSCE Station 33: Answer

A   There is asymmetry of and swelling in the left peritonsillar region, suggestive of quinsy.

B   ◆ Ear pain due to the effect on the glossopharyngeal nerve
   ◆ Inability to open the jaw due to the effect on the pterygoid muscles
   ◆ Difficulty swallowing
   ◆ Pain on swallowing
   ◆ Muffled voice

C   ◆ Drainage of the abscess via needle/incision, usually performed under local anaesthetic
   ◆ Antibiotics – usually penicillin with or without anaerobic cover
   ◆ Analgesia
   ◆ Abscess tonsillectomy – a controversial treatment, and many prefer to perform interval tonsillectomy after the quinsy has resolved

D   These complications are all caused by extension of inflammation to surrounding structures, notably the larynx and parapharyngeal space:

   ◆ respiratory obstruction/airway compromise
   ◆ parapharyngeal abscess
   ◆ meningitis
   ◆ cavernous sinus thrombosis
   ◆ brain abscess
   ◆ internal jugular vein thrombosis
   ◆ erosion of carotid artery
   ◆ invasion of parotid.

OSCE Station 34: Question

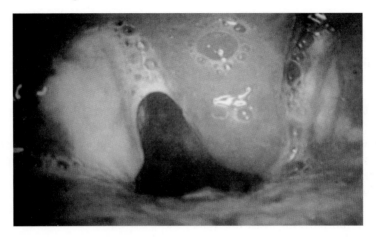

A This patient with tonsillitis has a diagnosis of glandular fever. What feature in the photograph is suggestive of this?

B What test may confirm the diagnosis?

C What virus is responsible for this infection?

D What advice should be given to the patient on discharge, and why?

OSCE Station 34: Answer

A The photograph shows evidence of fibrinous exudate covering the tonsils, which suggests infectious mononucleosis, or glandular fever.

B A Paul–Bunnell test (demonstration of heterophile antibodies in the serum) may be positive.

C The Epstein–Barr virus is the organism responsible.

D The patient should avoid contact sports for 2–3 months, as the virus may cause hepatosplenomegaly and leave these organs more prone to damage through trauma. Treatment with amoxicillin should be avoided, as an allergic-type rash may develop – penicillin should be used instead.

OSCE Station 35: Question

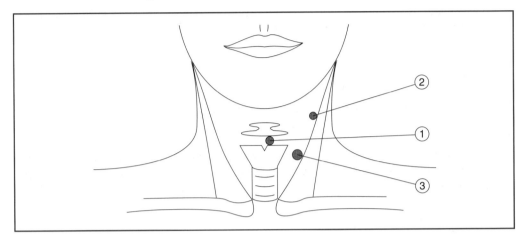

Describe the position the lumps shown in the figure would occupy. Name one feature of each lump that would be obvious on examination. Which groups of patients mostly present with each lump?

OSCE Station 35: Answer

1   Thyroglossal cyst – usually very close to, or on the midline, anywhere from the tongue base to the thyroid gland. Examination shows a lump that moves with tongue protrusion and swallowing. Patients are usually young children.

2   Chemodectoma – on the anterior border of sternocleidomastoid in the area of the carotid bifurcation at the superior edge of the thyroid cartilage. The lump will be pulsatile and will move in an antero-posterior plane, but not up or down. Patients may be of any age, but the problem is commonest in those who live at high altitudes.

3   Branchial cyst – on the anterior border of the sternocleidomastoid around the level of the cricoid cartilage (although it may be a little higher or lower than this). The lump usually transilluminates on examination. Patients are usually in their third decade.

OSCE Station 36: Question

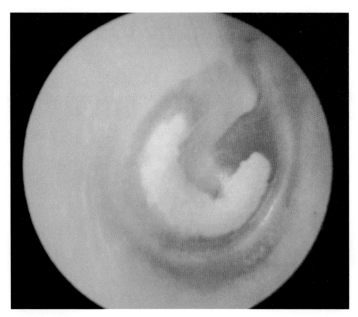

This is a figure of a tympanic membrane.

A   What is the diagnosis?

B   What might the audiogram be expected to show?

OSCE Station 36: Answer

A   Tympanosclerosis: calcareous deposits on the tympanic membrane due to the formation of an exudate and consequent repair, with fibroblast invasion, collagen synthesis and calcification.

B   Very large tympanosclerosis plaques may cause conductive hearing loss, but in this case a normal audiogram is present, as the tympanic membrane still shows enough compliance to transmit sound.

OSCE Station 37: Question

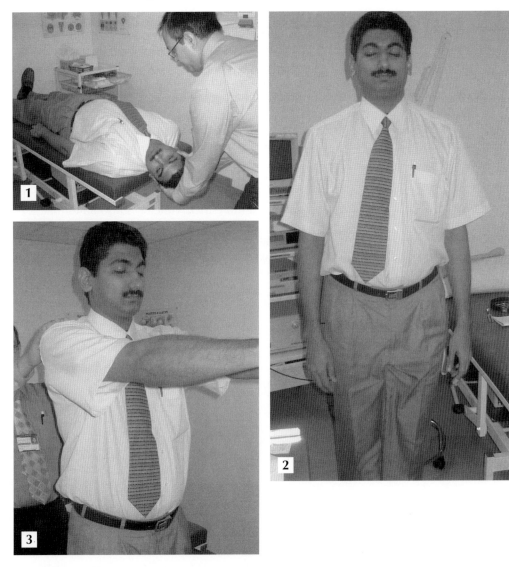

A   Name the manoeuvres/tests shown in the figures which are involved in the diagnosis and treatment of vertigo. In each case state briefly what information the test may provide.

B   What is Epley's manoeuvre?

OSCE Station 37: Answer

A 1 Dix–Hallpike test – this test may precipitate positional vertigo. The patient is positioned sitting on a bed, and their head is rotated to 45° to the side. The patient is then laid backwards with their head over the edge of the bed, at approximately 30° below the horizontal. The patient is asked if symptoms are provoked and they are observed for nystagmus, and then they are returned to the vertical. Precipitation of symptoms indicates a possible diagnosis of benign paroxysmal positional vertigo.

2 Romberg's test – the patient stands with feet together, eyes closed, and arms by the side. Peripheral vestibular lesions produce a tendency to fall to the side of the lesion.

3 Unterberger's test – the patient steps on the spot with the eyes closed and the arms extended. A rotation of more than 40° indicates labyrinthine pathology on that side. Forwards or backwards displacement of more than 1 metre is also abnormal.

B This is a sequence of movements designed to displace otoconic deposits in the inner ear. It provides a 'cure' for benign paroxysmal positional vertigo in 80% of patients when correctly performed.

OSCE Station 38: Question

The following results are observed in a 50-year-old woman, who is not on any medication.

- T_4 **30.0** (normal range 7–25 pmol/L)
- TSH **0.1** (normal range 0.3–4 mU/L)

A   What is the diagnosis?

B   Name three symptoms that may be present.

C   Name three signs that may be present.

D   What blood test may be used to confirm the diagnosis?

OSCE Station 38: Answer

A Thyrotoxicosis, caused by Graves' disease, due to stimulation of the TSH receptors by IgG antibodies. It leads to an increase in thyroid hormones, and a consequent reduction in TSH secretion by a feedback mechanism.

B Thyrotoxicosis may be accompanied by:

- diarrhoea
- weight loss
- heat intolerance
- anxiety
- palpitations
- sweating.

C Thyrotoxicosis may cause:

- exophthalmos
- lid lag
- lid retraction
- chemosis
- oculomotor paralysis
- goitre
- tachycardia or atrial fibrillation
- tremor
- pretibial myxoedema.

D The patient can be tested for anti-thyroglobulin antibodies – their presence indicates Graves' disease.

OSCE Station 39: Question

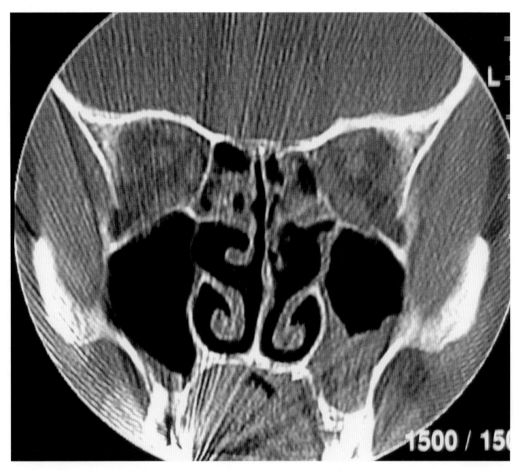

A   Name the two sinuses shown on this CT scan segment.

B   What pathology does the CT scan show?

OSCE Station 39: Answer

A   The ethmoid and maxillary sinuses.

B   There is sinus disease in the left maxillary sinus, which may represent an air–fluid level. There is also thickening of both ethmoid sinuses. Both of these changes signify chronic sinus disease.

OSCE Station 40: Question

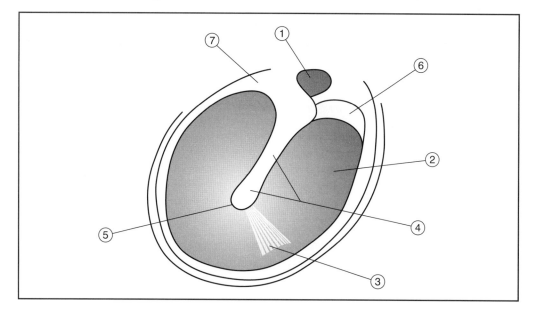

Name the structures marked in this drawing of the right tympanic membrane.

SECTION 5

OSCE Station 40: Answer

1   Pars flaccida

2   Pars tensa

3   Light reflex

4   Handle of malleus

5   Umbo

6   Anterior malleolar fold

7   Posterior malleolar fold

OSCE Station 41: Question

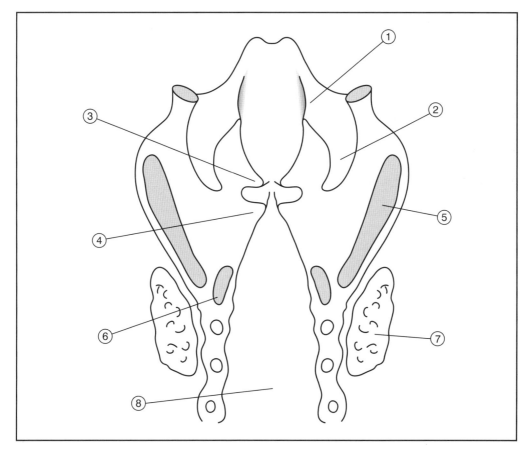

Name the structures marked in the diagram.

SECTION 5

OSCE Station 41: Answer

1   Aryepiglottic fold

2   Pyriform fossa

3   Vestibular/false cords

4   Vocal/true cords

5   Thyroid cartilage

6   Cricoid cartilage

7   Thyroid gland

8   Trachea

OSCE Station 42: Question

A Describe the characteristics of a classic attack of Ménière's disease.

B Describe the classic audiometric finding on a pure tone audiogram in established Ménière's disease.

C Name three long-term medical treatments that have been suggested for Ménière's disease.

OSCE Station 42: Answer

A Patients with true Ménière's disease have intermittent attacks of deafness, tinnitus and vertigo which last a few hours. The attacks may be preceded by a prodromal phase, which is often a feeling of fullness in the ear. Between attacks the patient is usually normal in the early stages of the disease.

B Established disease may produce a normal audiogram, but classically the finding is of a low-frequency, unilateral, sensorineural hearing loss.

C ◆ Salt restriction
   ◆ Fluid restriction
   ◆ Betahistine
   ◆ Diuretics

Question Index

Note: This index is only to the questions in this book and is by question number.

E: denotes Extended Matching questions, and M: denotes Multiple True/False questions

Index

Please note: page numbers in **bold** type refer to figures; those in *italics,* to material in boxes or tables.

INDEX

INDEX

laryngeal carcinoma 171, 214
  paralysis 121, 174, 218
voice 96–97
  hoarseness 171, 214, 244–245
  muffled 314
  post-surgery changes 148, 192, 264
voice hearing testing 29

W

Waldeyer's ring 119
Walshingham's forceps **249**, 250
warfarin therapy 132, 133, 183, 184
  epistaxis and 146, 191

Warthin's tumour 108, 172, 173, 216
wax, ear canal 38, 142, 188, 204
Weber's test 29–30, 135, 162, 185, 202,
  228, **230**
Wegener's granulomatosis 62–63, 168,
  209
  septal perforation 168, 210
Willis' paracusis 189
wounds (surgical) *10*, 12–14

X

X-ray (plain) 21, 144, 160, 190, 198

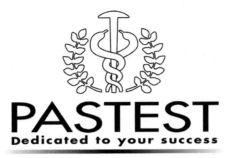

PASTEST
Dedicated to your success

PasTest has been publishing books for doctors for over 30 years. Our extensive experience means that we are always one step ahead when it comes to knowledge of current trends and content of the Royal College exams.

We use only the best authors and lecturers, many of whom are Consultants and Royal College Examiners, which enables us to tailor our books and courses to meet your revision needs. We incorporate feedback from candidates to ensure that our books are continually improved.

This commitment to quality ensures that students who buy a PasTest book or attend a PasTest course achieve successful exam results.

Delivery to your Door
With a busy lifestyle, nobody enjoys walking to the shops for something that may or may not be in stock. Let us take the hassle and deliver direct to your door. We will despatch your book within 24 hours of receiving your order.

How to Order:

www.pastest.co.uk
To order our books safely and securely online, shop online at our website.

Telephone: +44 (0)1565 752000
Fill out the order form as a helpful prompt and have your credit card to hand when you call.

PasTest Ltd, FREEPOST, Knutsford, WA16 7BR
Send your completed order form with your cheque (made payable to **PasTest Ltd**) and debit or credit card details to the above address. (Please complete your address details on the reverse of the cheque.)

Fax: +44 (0)1565 650264
Fax your completed order form with your debit or credit card details.

Pastest courses

PASTEST: the key to exam success, the key to your future

PasTest is dedicated to helping doctors to pass their professional examinations. We have 30 years of specialist experience in medical education and over 3000 doctors attend our revision courses each year.

Experienced lecturers:
Many of our lecturers are also examiners and teach in a lively and interesting way in order to:

◆ reflect current trends in exams
◆ give plenty of mock exam practice
◆ provide valuable advice on exam technique

Outstanding accelerated learning:
Our up-to-date and relevant course material includes MCQs, colour slides, X-rays, ECGs, EEGs, clinical cases, data interpretations, mock exams, vivas and extensive course notes which provide:

◆ hundreds of high quality questions with detailed answers and explanations
◆ succinct notes, diagrams and charts

Personal attention:
Active participation is encouraged on these courses, so in order to give personal tuition and to answer individual questions our course numbers are limited. Book early to avoid disappointment.

Choice of courses:
PasTest has developed a wide range of high quality interactive courses in different cities around the UK to suit your individual needs.

What other candidates have said about our courses:
'Absolutely brilliant – I would not have passed without it! Thank you.'
Dr Charitha Rajapakse, London.

'Excellent, enjoyable, extremely hard work but worth every penny.'
Dr Helen Binns, Oxford.

For further details contact:
PasTest Ltd, Egerton Court, Parkgate Estate
Knutsford, Cheshire WA16 8DX, UK.
Telephone: 01565 752000 Fax: 01565 650264
e-mail: courses@pastest.co.uk website: www.pastest.co.uk